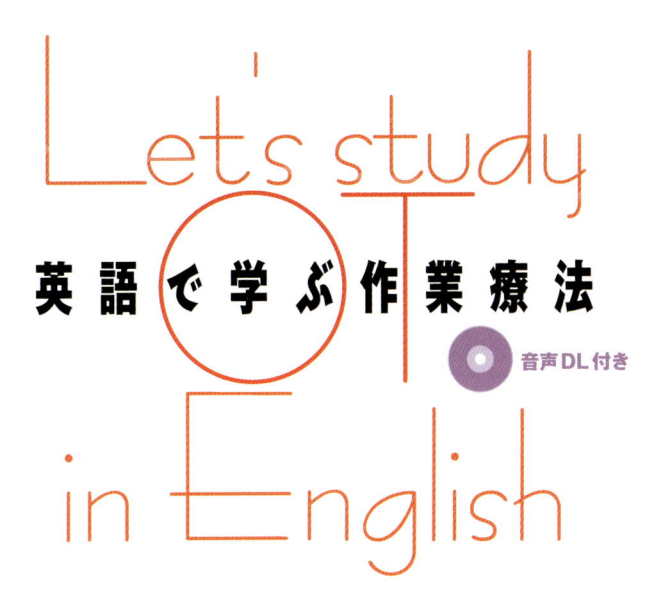

Let's study OT in English
英語で学ぶ作業療法

音声DL付き

[監修]
菊池恵美子
（帝京平成大学 健康メディカル学部 作業療法学科 教授）

[著]
山内ひさえ
（作業療法士・保健科学博士）

吉川ひろみ
（県立広島大学 保健福祉学部 作業療法学科 教授）

Peter Kenneth Howell
（広島大学 外国語教育研究センター 准教授）

＊監修・著者の所属、職位は初版発行時のものです。

『英語で学ぶ作業療法　Let's Study OT in English』音声ダウンロード

本書の音声データ(MP3 形式)を以下の URL よりダウンロードいただけます。
(ファイルは ZIP 形式で圧縮されていますので、別途、解凍ソフトが必要です。)
なお、音声データにつきましては、初版発行時に録音したもので、
一部テキストと音声が異なる場合がございます。
ご不便をおかけいたしますが、その旨ご了承ください。

https://cbr-pub.com/book/022-download.html

まえがき

　本書の企画は、筆者が首都大学東京を退官後に着任した帝京平成大学において「現代英語」を担当することになったことがきっかけでした。この「現代英語」は全学必修科目で、他学部も合わせると3,000名を超える学生を25名前後の小クラスに分け、英語の教員免許がない教師も担当するというユニークなものでした。

　英語の講義は、留学の経験からイメージが湧きましたが、困ったのは教材です。保健医療職を目指す学生向けの教本も市販されてはいますが、作業療法学生のニーズに合うものが見当たりません。なければ創りたいと、旧知のCBR三輪敏社長にご相談したところ、今までにないような本ができるのであれば、とご賛同を頂きました。幸い、執筆者には学部・院を現・首都大学東京で学ばれた山内ひさえ氏とウェスタンミシガン大学で修士号を取得された県立広島大学OT学科長・教授の吉川ひろみ氏のご協力を得ることができました。

　前述の如く、本書は英語教材としてスタートしております。しかし、作成のプロセスを通して、タイトルが『英語で学ぶ作業療法』であるように、これは「基礎作業療法学」や「作業療法評価学」の副読本として、学生に作業療法のイメージを持たせ、基本的な作業療法プロセスを学ばせる教材として使えるのでは、との思いが強くなりました。

　本書は全5章27項から構成されています。全編を通して、主人公2人の会話を主体に、辞書がなくても読める平易な英語表現になるよう工夫を凝らしてあります。第1章は作業療法士への動機や学生への講義について、第2章と3章は、臨床実習を舞台にして学生が戸惑いがちなシーンやテーマを取り上げました。第4章は症例を挙げながらICFやCMOP、MOHOの理論およびクリニカルリーズニ

ングと関連付けて解説しています。さらに第5章では、アリソン・ウィックス世界作業科学研究会会長のご助言を得て、吉川氏による「occupation（作業）」とその概念が力説されています。氏のメッセージ「英語で作業療法を語ることができるようになれば、世界の作業療法コミュニティに参加することができます。海外の作業療法士と話して感じるのは、可視化しにくい曖昧な仕事をしているという私たちの類似性です。それでもみんな作業療法の魅力にとりつかれています。Sharing an occupational therapy perspective（作業療法の視点の共有）に向かって一歩を踏み出しませんか。」を、お伝えしておきたいと思います。

　学生諸子には、主人公に自らを重ね合わせることで、作業療法への動機付けから卒業まで、共に成長しながら学んで欲しいと思います。また、養成校の先生方には本書の活用を通して、日本語では教えにくい「作業」や学生が戸惑いがちなテーマをさらに発展させて頂き、ご批判頂ければと思います。

　最後になりましたが、英語の監修をして頂いたピーター・ハウエル氏、付属CDにご出演頂いたネイティブスピーカーの方々、英語会議通訳者の姉崎祐治氏、写真撮影をご許可頂いた帝京平成大学学長、撮影に協力してくれた作業療法学科教員と学生有志、そして何より、本書の企画から完成までをきめ細かにサポートして頂いたCBRの三輪敏社長と長沢慎吾様に心から感謝申し上げます。

　　　　　　　　　　　　　　　　　2011年3月　　菊池恵美子

Contents

| Prologue | 001 |

Chapter 1 — *Fundamental study for occupational therapy*

§1	Why do you want to become an occupational therapist?	002
§2	What do you have to study to be an occupational therapist?	006
§3	What does occupation mean?	010

Chapter 2 — *Clinical training : Assessment*

§1	A greeting and explanation of occupational therapy	014
§2	Sharing information with medical team members	018
§3	Interview	022
§4	Physical functions	026
§5	Psychological functions	030
§6	Higher brain dysfunction	034

Chapter 3 — *Completion of assessment and treatment*

| §1 | Conference for setting a goal and program in occupational therapy | 038 |

§2	Occupational therapy for physical dysfunction	**042**
§3	Occupational therapy for mental disorders	**046**
§4	Occupational therapy for developmental disabilities	**050**
§5	Occupational therapy for elderly people	**054**
§6	Community-based occupational therapy	**058**

Chapter 4 — *Client-centered occupational therapy*

⟨*Mr. Okada's case : CVA*⟩

§1	ICF : International Classification of Functioning, Disability and Health	**062**
§2	A practice based on CMOP (Canadian Model of Occupational Performance)	**066**
§3	Clinical reasoning to think in action	**070**

⟨*Mrs. Hara's case : RA*⟩

§4	A practice based on MOHO (Model of Human Occupation)	**074**
§5	Joint protection for ADL and IADL	**078**
§6	Environmental modification	**082**

Chapter 5 — *Fundamental concepts*

§1	Occupation	**086**
§2	Engagement in occupation	**090**

§3	Occupational justice	094
§4	Inclusion	098
§5	Rehabilitation	102
§6	Health promotion	106

| | Epilogue | 113 |

Appendix — The Japanese welfare system / Globalization

Services and Supports for Persons with Disabilities Act	114
Long-term Care Insurance Law	115
Act for the Mental Health and Welfare of Persons with Mental Disorders	116
Act on Employment Promotion etc. of Persons with Disabilities	117
Study and work abroad	118
WFOT (World Federation of Occupational Therapists)	119
JOCV (Japan Overseas Cooperation Volunteers)	120

| Glossary | 121 |

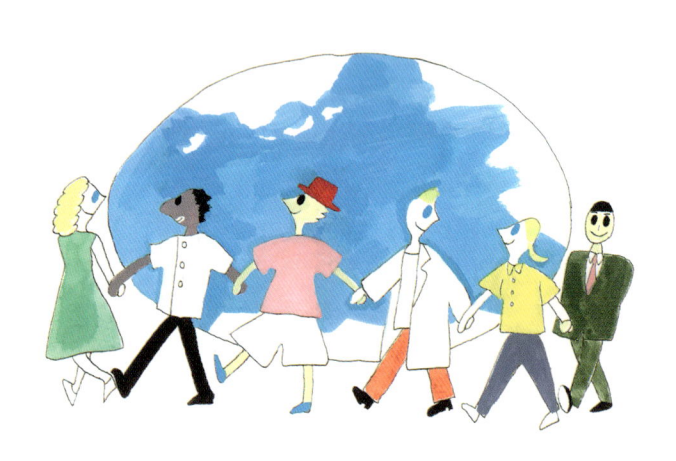

Prologue

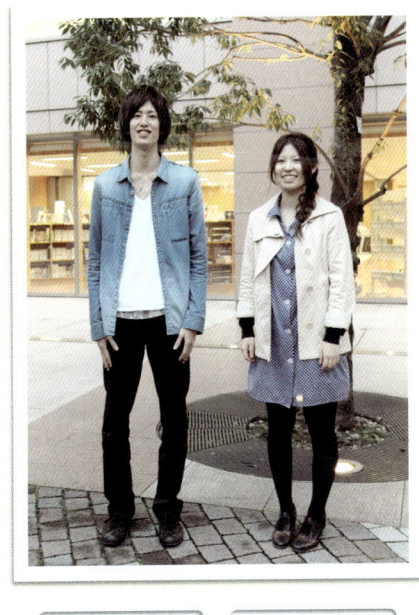

Taku *Maki*

Spring
A new school year begins. A boy meets a girl. They are classmates in the department of occupational therapy (OT).

The boy's name is Taku. He has a sense of justice and humor, and has a tendency to act without much consideration. He wants to become a good occupational therapist.

Maki is an honest, kind, and hardworking student. Sometimes she is too rational to feel sympathy with people. In particular she wants to work for persons with disabilities and for society in general.

Fundamental study for occupational therapy

> Hello.
> I am Taku. I am a student in the OT department.

> Hi. My name is Maki.
> I'm in the OT department, too.
> I know you. You are always cheerful.

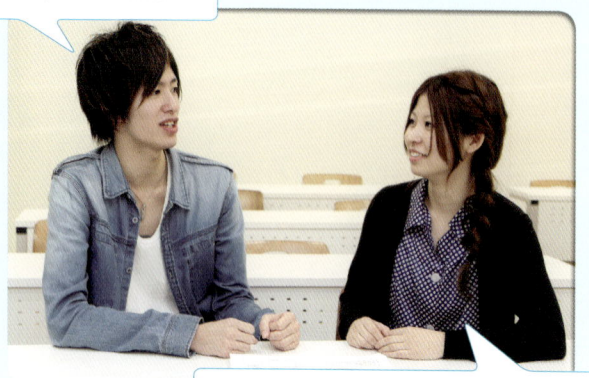

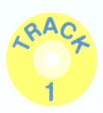

TRACK 1

Section 1

Why do you want to become an occupational therapist?

Objective

To explain your motivation to become an OT

Taku is waiting for a chance to talk with Maki.
At last he introduces himself. And he asks her why she wants to become an OT, because he wants to know her more.

§1 Why do you want to become an occupational therapist?

Taku: Why do you want to become an occupational therapist?

Maki: Because I want to work with people with disabilities.

Taku: You found something worthwhile, didn't you?

Maki: Yes. My grandmother suffered from strokes, so she had some physical and mental disorders. And she had dementia. I saw some physical therapists and occupational therapists at that time. So I became interested in OT.

Taku: Tell me the reason why you're interested in OT?

Maki: When the first stroke happened to my grandmother, she couldn't do anything by herself. We were confused, and felt anxious. But an occupational therapist enabled her to do some activities, for example activities of daily life, painting, going out to meet good friends. Those kinds of activities helped my grandmother to be cheerful again. I want to make people with disabilities happy, too.

Taku: You seem to be a really nice person.

Maki: How about you? Why do you want to become an OT?

OT:作業療法
Occupational Therapy
あるいは作業療法士
Occupational Therapist

OTR:有資格作業療法士
Registered Occupational Therapist

RNはRegistered Nurse、RPTはRegistered Physical Therapist。ROTとしないのは「腐った」という意味の語となるのを避けるためである。

OTS:作業療法学生
Occupational Therapy Student

PWD(Persons with disabilities):
病気や怪我による機能障害だけでなく、加齢、災害、戦争などにより、日常の活動や社会参加の障害を経験している人々。

stroke:
病気、発作に襲われること。特に脳卒中。

dementia:
認知症

Enabling:
できるようになること。可能化。Enabling occupation（作業の可能化）は作業療法の目標である。

Chapter 1

Fundamental study for occupational therapy

Taku : Well first, I want to help my friends who have serious disabilities.

Maki : What kind of disabilities do they have?

Taku : One of them can't stand and hasn't been able to use his right hand throughout his whole life. Another is bedridden. I was in hospital for several months because of an accident in my second year of high school. We became good friends after sharing the same hospital room.

Maki : I feel sorry for your friends.

Taku : Whenever I thought about their future, I felt hopeless. Then unexpectedly, they were discharged. One of them could even return to work. The other one, who is still bedridden, can live comfortably in a room set up for him. They say OTs are very useful to help re-construct their lives. If an OT can give hope to people with disabilities, I want to try the job.

Maki : We have something in common. Hey Kana, how about you?

Kana, a friend of Maki, joins them

Kana : Why do I want to be an OT? To get a national qualification as a medical expert.

Taku : That sounds like a nice plan.

---

be bedridden:
寝たきり

can live comfortably in a room set up for him:
彼の身体機能に合わせ、彼が可能な限り快適にかつ自立した生活を送れるように環境調整した部屋。

to re-construct their life:
彼の生活や人生を再構築する。

national qualification:
国家資格

§1 Why do you want to become an occupational therapist?

What is the job of an OT?

In 1964, a law for physical therapists and occupational therapists was established. Before the law, activities such as therapy and vocational training were used in psychiatry or in education for children with disabilities by care staff, teachers, and so on. After the law, occupational therapists became one of a number of medical rehabilitation team members.

At the present time, the role of occupational therapist is expanding from the medical setting to health, welfare, and education. Occupational therapists are working in hospitals, welfare centers, government offices, rehabilitation centers, home-visit services, day care centers, care facilities for older people, nursing homes, schools, and businesses.

The World Federation of Occupational Therapists (WFOT) revised the definition of occupational therapy in 2004. Occupational therapy is a profession concerned with promoting health and well being through occupation. The primary goal of occupational therapy is to enable people to participate in the activities of everyday life.
(WFOT: definition of OT)
〈http://www.wfot.org/office_files/DEFINITIONS%20-%20DRAFT9%202009-2010.pdf〉

Question

Why do you want to be an occupational therapist?

Chapter 1

Fundamental study for occupational therapy

> There are too many subjects to study.

> I am not good at statistics.

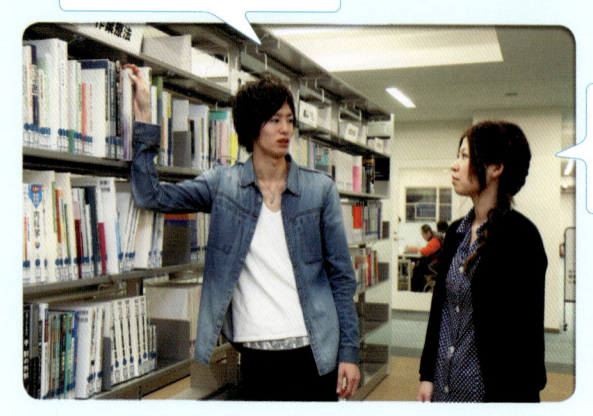

TRACK 2

Section 2

What do you have to study to be an occupational therapist?

Objective

To explain what you have to study

Taku is frustrated by the many subjects he has to study. He is not a hard worker, but professors teach him many things everyday. He is not sure what you have to study to become a good OT.

§2 What do you have to study to be an occupational therapist?

Taku : I'm worried I might fail the anatomy and physiology examinations.

Maki : Don't worry. It's not easy for any student.

Taku : I don't know whether I can memorize the names of all the bones, muscles and nerves.

Maki : If you can't remember them, you can't understand functions. Anyway we must study little by little everyday.

Taku : I know. But I'm tired of studying complicated subjects.

Maki : We have to stick at it. After studying basic medicine, we will move on to clinical medicine.

Taku : I have a problem with statistics too. I failed it last year. So now, I feel I'm poor at statistical thinking.

Maki : I'm not good at statistics either.

Taku : That's a relief.

Maki : What do you mean?

---

anatomy:
解剖学

physiology:
生理学

rudimentary (basic) medicine:
基礎医学

kinesiology:
運動学

orthopedics:
整形外科 (学)

clinical medicine:
臨床医学

statistics:
統計学
権威者の主張や臨床家のカンで行われる医療に対して、実際に治療効果があったという証拠に基づいた医療 (evidence-based medicine: EBM) が推奨されている。EBMでは臨床データを分析した研究論文を理解するために、統計学の知識が必須である。

Fundamental study for occupational therapy

Taku : I feel better knowing you are weak in statistics like me.

Maki : OK. Are you feeling better now?

Taku : I think so. So let's stop talking about subjects we hate. What subject do you like or are you good at?

Maki : I am good at practical occupational therapy. For example, making devices, woodwork, ceramic art, weaving, handicrafts, painting, etc.. What subject do you like?

Taku : I am interested in learning about the relationship between disablement and environment. Do you remember the professor said that a person's occupational performance depends on his or her environment?

Maki : When we learned house modifications for people using wheelchairs, I was surprised that occupational therapists can be involved in so many kinds of things.

Taku : I feel like studying now. Thank you.

人の機能と環境:
医療の中で発展した作業療法は、解剖学や生理学など、人の構造や機能の学習を基本としてきた。しかし、機能が十分に発揮されるためには環境を考慮する必要がある。どの作業がどのようにできることが健康なのかを考えるためには、人の機能だけでなく、環境を知り環境に関わらなければならない。

§2 *What do you have to study to be an occupational therapist?*

The education of occupational therapists

OT students have to study many subjects.

Firstly, the basic field aims to establish a basis of scientific thinking and to know about human beings and human life.

Secondly, the specialized field has two components.

One is the special basic field containing rudimentary medicine, and clinical medicine. Rudimentary medicine includes anatomy, physiology, pathology, human development, and kinesiology. Clinical medicine includes internal medicine, orthopedics, psychiatry, neurology, rehabilitation medicine, and gerontology.

The other is the special field of occupational therapy including basic occupational therapy, evaluation and treatment for occupational therapy, community-based occupational therapy and clinical training.

Why do OT students have to study such diverse subjects? Because occupation depends on the performance capacity of physical and mental function, the relationship between person and environment. So occupational therapists must have a proper and deep understanding about human life.

Question

What subjects do you have to learn and why?

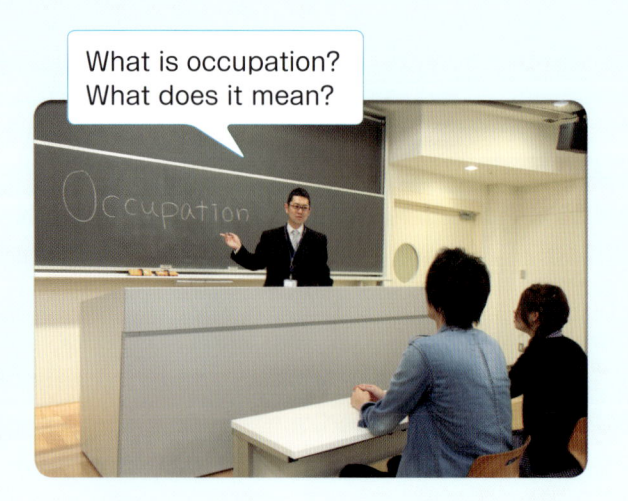

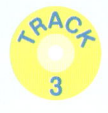

Chapter 1 — *Fundamental study for occupational therapy*

> What is occupation? What does it mean?

TRACK 3

Section 3

What does occupation mean?

Objective

To explain occupational state

Taku and Maki will go to clinical practice next month. They apply themselves closely to preparation and review. Now Professor Kusaka asks a question on a fundamental element of occupational therapy.

§3 What does occupation mean?

In occupational therapy intervention class

Kusaka : Have you ever thought why our job is called occupational therapy?

All students : .... *(silence)*

Kusaka : Taku, what does occupation mean?

Taku : I don't know. Can I check the dictionary?

Kusaka : Sure.

Taku : Occupation means action, state, or period of occupying or being occupied, a job or profession, a way of spending time.

Kusaka : So, how does that relate to our job?

Taku : All of those things are relevant to occupational therapy.

Kusaka : Maki, what do you think?

Maki : I think the definition is about a person's situation.

Kusaka : Situation?

OTの説明:

かつて、作業療法の説明では、occupationを使う代わりにactivity、taskといった語が使われてきた。気晴らし的活動(diversional activity)、治療的活動(therapeutic activity)、目的活動(purposeful activity)がよく使われてきた。しかし1960年前後に登場した作業行動(occupational behavior)理論、1980年に発表され改訂が続いている人間作業モデル(model of human occupation)など作業療法理論が発展し、作業(occupation)という語が多く使われるようになった。1989年には、作業を探究する学問として作業科学(occupational science)も誕生した。

→Chapter 5参照

Chapter 1 — Fundamental study for occupational therapy

Maki : For example, doing something, the state they're in, the context…maybe occupation explains individual situation.

Kusaka : That's a good point. Well Taku, what do you think is meant by "spending time"?

Taku : Does it mean a pastime?

Kusaka : It's not the only way of spending time. All activities are spending time. It also means ways of living. All life on earth has a unique, specific and particular style of life, but human beings are special. Human life is made up of countless choices. How do you make choices in your life?

Taku : Well, I guess I choose to do or not to do something by making priorities. I decide by using my experience, desire, and circumstances.

Kusaka : Exactly. The result is that you yourself decide how to spend time in your life.

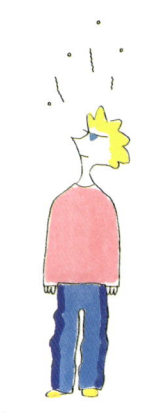

I have nothing to do.

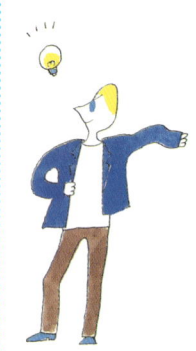

I have something I want to do.

§3 What does occupation mean?

What does occupation mean?

Kielhofner, an American scholar of occupational therapy, states that human occupation is a dynamic system which is composed of volitional processes, habituation and environment.

Can you imagine what life would be like if you could not make any decision by yourself? You would surely lose a lot of life's pleasure, and you might not even find life worth living. If you have to travel everyday, maybe your life would be uncomfortable. If your environment were poor, maybe you wouldn't feel any satisfaction in life.

People want to live their own life as they want. For this purpose, you decide what, where, when and how to do things. That makes you have a unique pattern of daily living, work, friendship, leisure and other things that are important for you.

Occupation defines your own way of life.

Question

What does occupation mean?

Chapter 2

Clinical training : Assessment

> Nice to meet you. I am an OT student.

> Nice meeting of you. What is OT?

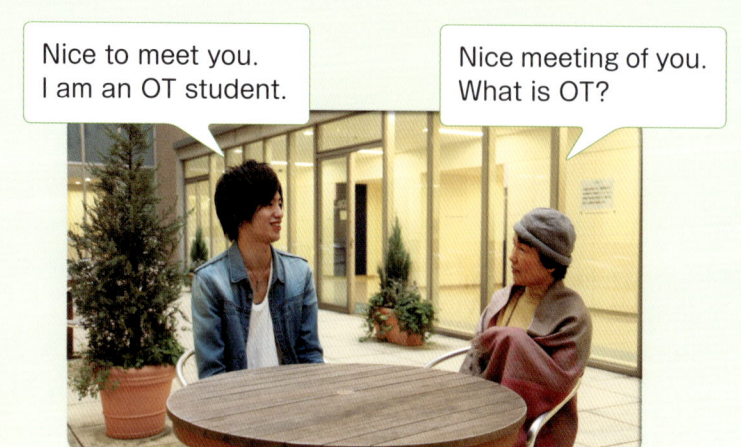

TRACK 4

Section 1

A greeting and explanation of occupational therapy

Objective

To introduce yourself and explain OT to clients

Taku has started clinical training in a general hospital. OTS must introduce themselves and explain OT to several different clients.

At first Taku thought it was easy. But now he is at a loss how to explain the OT's role.

§1 A greeting and explanation of occupational therapy

Supervisor (SV): This is the first day of your training. Before anything else, let's exchange greetings and explain occupational therapy (OT). How would you explain OT?

Taku: Well, occupational therapy is a treatment which uses handicrafts, arts, playing games, activities of daily living, housework, and other activities. It is mainly effective for people who have mental or physical trouble to help them recover applied operational capability or social adjustment capability.

SV: All right. Let's try and explain it to a client.

In a hospital room. A male patient, Mr. Okada, is lying down on his bed. He has suffered a stroke, and he has severe right hemi-paralysis.

Taku: Hello. I'm an occupational therapy student. My name is Taku. Nice to meet you.

Okada: Nice to meet you too. What kind of student did you say?

Taku: An occupational therapy student. Occupational therapy is a kind of treatment with some activities for people with disabilities.

Okada: What kind of activities? How can you treat me?

Physical Therapists and Occupational Therapists Act:
理学療法士および作業療法士法
第二条2項では、
「作業療法とは、身体又は精神に障害のある者に対し、主としてその応用的動作能力又は社会的適応能力の回復を図るため、手芸、工作その他の作業を行なわせることをいう」
（1965年）
と定義し、主に巧緻性、ADL（日常生活動作）、上肢の運動機能、高次脳機能の向上を目的とする。

SV:Supervisor
臨地（床）指導者

OTの説明:
OTの社会認知度を高めるために、海外では次のようなキャッチコピーがある。
・Living life to its fullest
・Skills for the job of living
・Health by doing
・Towards meaningful life

015

Clinical training : Assessment

Taku : For example, handicrafts, art…and self-care, activities of daily living, and other activities you need.

Okada : I need to get back to my job as soon as possible. Can you treat my right hand? I can't do anything if it doesn't get better.

Taku : Ah, I see. Let me think about your needs.

Taku meets a female patient, Mrs. Kawai, and her husband, Mr. Kawai. She is suffering from Parkinson's disease.

Mr. Kawai : Handicrafts and art? She doesn't like those kinds of things. She can take care of herself except for some activities like taking a bath. But I can help and we will request a home helper. So we don't need housework training. We need other treatment such as walking and preventing progression of dementia.

Taku : Some activities are effective in slowing the progress of dementia.

After going out of the room

SV : Well, you're the therapist in charge. Do you think they've understood occupational therapy?

作業療法の種目と目的のわかりにくさ：
作業療法は、さまざまな姿勢でのバランス機能、目的にあった上肢の協調性や巧緻性、状況判断し適応的に目的を遂行する能力などを、家庭や学校、職場、公共の場で発揮できるよう訓練する。
しかし「そのために手工芸を行います」と説明しても理解してもらいにくい。例えば、身体を大きく動かすゲームや、編み物や革細工をするとき、どれほどの機能が刺激され訓練されているのかを理解してもらうことが重要である。

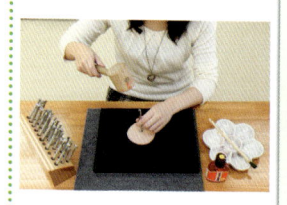

OTが使う作業：
作業療法が日本に導入された1950年代後半は、治療手段としての作業の利用が注目されていた時代だった。現在は「手段としての作業 (occupation as means)」だけではなく、その作業をすることそのものが生活の一部を構成する「目的としての作業 (occupation as end)」も重視されている。

§1 A greeting and explanation of occupational therapy

Why is it difficult to explain OT?

Is it difficult to explain OT? Yes! It is not easy for students but it's also difficult for many occupational therapists. But why? Possibly, the difficulty comes from the difference of opinion about occupation between occupational therapists and others.

Many occupations are common to people. Most of them are daily routine and universal activities. They are not special except for very special jobs like astronauts. Rehabilitation by occupation? Most ordinary people may think: What does that mean?

But occupational therapists are not looking at uniqueness or specialty of activities but at their meanings to individuals. This meaning signifies that every activity has its purpose for individual life. And the purpose can rescue people with disabilities from their disappointment.

If you need to explain OT to your client, you should tell them about the meaning of occupations that are very important for the client.

Question

Explain occupation and the OT's job?

Clinical training : Assessment

> I would like to know about Mrs.Wada.

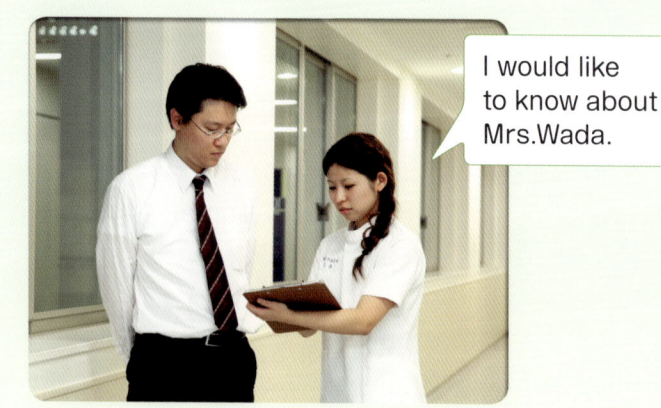

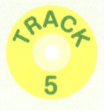

TRACK 5

Section 2

Sharing information with medical team members

Objective

How to collect and exchange information

Maki is instructed by her supervisor to collect information about a female patient who has had a stroke. The physician in charge of the patient has already approved the proposal to start occupational therapy for her. Now, her supervisor gives another instruction to exchange information about the patient with the hospital staff. Maki has a grandmother who suffered from a stroke, so she thinks that she already knows a lot about strokes.

§2 Sharing information with medical team members

SV : Maki, have you gathered information about Mrs. Wada, who was admitted to the hospital last week.

Maki : I check her medical record everyday.

SV : Do you understand that she's in the process of recovering from her stroke?

Maki : Yes. I learned about that in school. And my grandmother once suffered a stroke.

SV : Mm...also, you have to share information with nurses, doctors and physical therapists.

Maki : What information should I give them?

SV : Whatever they need.

With a nurse (Ns)

Ns : What do you want to know?

Maki : How is her consciousness and physical condition?

Ns : For her physical condition please check the medical records. You'll find the information you're looking for. Anything else?

Maki : How is her mental state?

Ns : She has just recovered consciousness. She finds it hard to face reality, and gets depressed.

情報の共有と交換:
医療・福祉の現場では情報は記録され共有される。しかし、すべてが記載されるわけではない。また、医師、看護師、PT、STなど、それぞれの専門職がそれぞれの視点からみた「重要な情報」が必ずしもOTが知りたいすべてではない。そこで直接に質問し、カンファレンスなどを利用して、情報を交換することが重要になる。

他職種に何を伝えるか:
「OTとして、他職種に伝えるべき情報は何か」と聞かれると、実習生や新人OTは戸惑うかもしれない。
OTが何をしているのかも当然だが、相手の仕事、例えば、医師は治療し回復させること、看護師は病棟でのケアや生活の管理である。その仕事の目的と内容に関係した情報を伝えていくことも必要である。

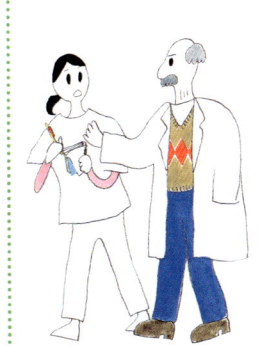

Clinical training : Assessment

Ns : So, when will you start occupational therapy with her? And where? Will you visit her or shall we take her to the OT room? What will you do first?

With a doctor (Dr)

Dr : Have you checked her medical records and prescription? Any questions?

Maki : Is there any special attention she needs?

Dr : Why don't you check the progress of recovery, and appearance of other symptoms?

With Mr. and Mrs. Wada

Maki : Before the stroke, what kind of life did she lead? Tell me about her job, hobbies, roles and anything important for her?

Mr. Wada : She's a teacher. Her hobbies are singing and travelling. What do you mean by roles? Will she get well soon?

Maki : ....

With SV

SV : So, was your knowledge from your grandmother's stroke useful? You have to learn two things. First, every patient has different symptoms and needs. Second, exchanging information should be mutually beneficial.

---

progress of recovery:
strokeの発作直後に脳の病変から起こった症状は段階的に決まったプロセスで回復していく。しかし、これはstrokeに限らずいくつもの疾患でみられる。

病名が同じでも…:
マキは、祖母も「stroke」だったから、ワダさんの症状についても自分は理解できるはずだと思い込んでいた。しかし、脳の発症部位によって起こる症状や後遺障害は人によって異なる。また発症部位だけでなく、さまざまな要因によっても異なる。

§2 Sharing information with medical team members

Collecting and exchanging information

Where is the important information?
Of course, it is in medical records, and other kinds of records taken by Dr, Ns, PT, ST, CP (clinical psychologists), SW (social workers) and so on. OT students have to read and understand those records.

OT students will be aware that some important information cannot be found in the records. Because each specialist has different points of view. In other words the roles of Dr, Ns, PT, ST and others are different from OT. So it is necessary to exchange information with all of them.

How do you exchange information with other staff?
You need to take a careful look at patients and exchange opinions with each other.

For example, if a patient always leaves food uneaten, a nurse would inform the occupational therapist. The therapist would try to find the cause, and let the nurse know the cause, for example, visual disorientation. Then they can cooperate and deal with the problem to improve visual function or to acquire new cognitive skills.

After all, to exchange information is to understand patients from several directions and to find how to cooperate with other staff.

Question

What information do you need to exchange? With whom? When?

Clinical training : Assessment

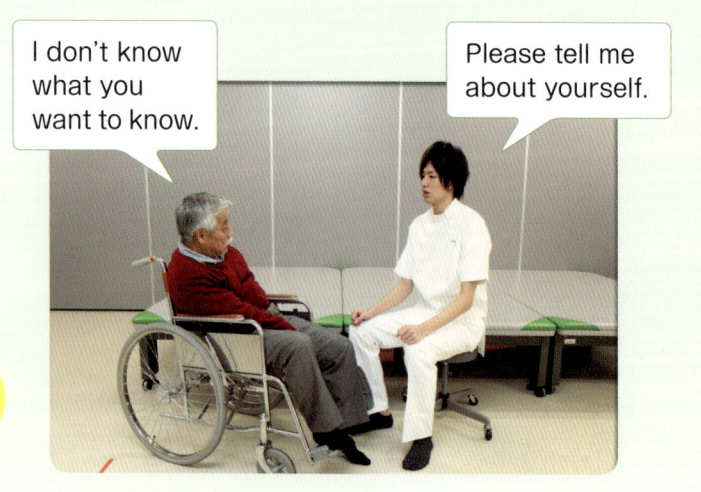

> I don't know what you want to know.

> Please tell me about yourself.

TRACK 6

Section 3
Interview

Objective

To learn how to interview clients

Taku is tackling a difficult subject.
It is to interview his clients. Why is it hard for him? He likes to talk to others, and of course with his clients, too. He was too optimistic in thinking that he could do interviews that would be sufficient for their OT assessment.
But now he starts to realize that an interview is different from a chat with his friends.

§3 Interview

SV : Taku, the purpose of interviews is to get patient information. I'd like you to arrange an interview with Mr. Okada.

In Mr. Okada's room

Taku : I'd like to hear from you about yourself and your disease. Is that OK with you?

Okada : OK. Where do you want to do it? Here?

Taku : Yes…ah, no. Just a moment please.

He looks around and sees other patients in the room.

Let's go to another room where it's quieter and more comfortable.

They go to another room. Firstly Taku takes a seat opposite Mr. Okada. But the SV signals with his eyes to change the seat to be at a right angle to Mr. Okada.

Taku : How are you feeling?

Okada : I'm having a very tough… tough time. I want to be free from the pain and paralysis…as I was before.

Taku : I hope we can help with that. Well, I have to know what practice I should give you. So let me ask some questions. What are the aspects of your life you want to get back?

Okada : Everything, of course.

Taku : I see. Now what is the most important thing for you：your job, your role or your hobbies?

Interviewの目的:
クライエントはひとりひとりが独自の存在であり、独特の価値観や人生観をもっている。作業療法を行ううえでInterviewの最も重要な目的は、クライエントの生活や人生に意味のある作業は何か、そしてその意味は何かという点を明らかにすることである。多くの場合、その意味とは重要な価値観や役割の反映であり、過去の成育歴やさまざまな経験に影響されている。

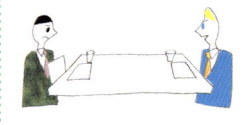

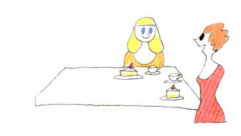

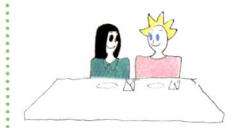

Clinical training : Assessment

Okada : Perfect recovery. Do you think I'll be left handicapped?

Taku : I can't predict exactly how your convalescence will go.

Okada : The highest priority for me is treatment of the paralysis. I want to move my body as before. Otherwise, my life is over.

Taku : Try not to look on the dark side of your situation. Even if you don't recover perfectly, you can still get back your health and life.

Okada : I don't think so. If I've lost the use of my body, I can't do my job, and might not be able to get a new job. How can I provide for my family? My role? I'm a father. I'm responsible for bringing up my children. Do you understand? I need recovery.

Taku : I understand very well.

After the interview

SV : Just after a stroke, many patients are like Mr. Okada. Before any questions, you should notice his anxiety. But you have learned the most important matters for him.

Next, you have to help him to give shape to his occupational goals.

Informed Consent:
十分な説明と同意

Try not to look on the dark side of your situation:
病気の直後には将来、とくに回復への不安や復職のことなどで悩んでしまいがちであるが、「悪いことばかり考えるな」と言われても、心はどうなるものではない。
作業療法に限らずリハビリテーションとは、「よいこと」や「未来の可能性」を実践の中でクライエントが感じ取れるよう配慮していくことも大切である。

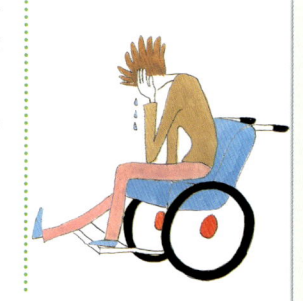

§3 *Interview*

What is a good interview?

Before an interview, there are some important things to do. The first is to collect sufficient information. The second is to arrange a place where your patient feels it is easy to talk, for example, a quiet, suitable, comfortable place with no one else around.

An interviewer must show respect and receptivity. What is the seating arrangement? Directly facing each other may make for a tense atmosphere. It is often said that sitting at a right angle to each other is better.

In an interview, you have to greet the patient and obtain their informed consent to be interviewed. Next, you should devise questions. You should use three types of questions— "closed", "open", and "if" questions— properly according to the situation. Sometimes you will get answers in non-verbal ways, for example posture and gestures. If patients say nothing, you should never force them to answer. It is most important that the occupational therapists should listen attentively and show sympathy, but never force their own opinion, analysis, suggestions into the interview. In OT, the purpose of an interview is to collect information about individual occupation, to establish a relationship with the patient, to confirm the individual problem and motivation and to reach consensus about what they should do.

Question

What should you do to make your interview successful?

Clinical training : Assessment

"Please keep your shoulder in external rotation."

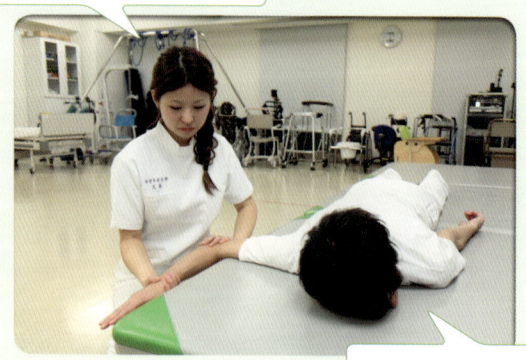

"External rotation…?"

TRACK 7

Section 4

Physical functions

Objective

To assess physical functions

Maki has acquired the skills required for assessment of physical functions. She practiced them very hard. However, she finds it difficult to get her patients to follow her instructions because her patients do not know technical terms. She is not confident about explaining things to her patients in simple words instead of technical terms.

§4 Physical functions

Maki assesses Mrs. Hara's range of motion of joints and muscle strength. She is suffering from rheumatoid arthritis (RA).

Maki : I'll check how far you can move your hand without pain and stiffness, and how strong your muscles are. Please move as I say. Stop if you feel pain, stiffness or anything uncomfortable.

Hara : OK. That sounds easy.

Maki : So, please lie on your back on the bed. First, I'll check your shoulder movement. I'll hold your right upper arm. Please raise your arm. OK. I'll put your arm down. One more time. Please raise your right upper arm against my resistance. OK.

Another client
Maki assesses Mrs. Wada who has had a stroke. She has paralysis on the left side of her body.

Maki : I'll check your paralysis. I'll bend your left arm at the elbow and put your left hand near your ear. Next, please bend your right arm at the elbow. I'll grasp your wrist. Please bend your right arm against my resistance. OK. Next, please move your left hand down to the right side of your waist.

Wada : What's wrong with my arm? Why can't I move my arm and leg at will?

Maki : Because of the stroke, the messages from your brain aren't getting through to the muscle. Paralysis after a stroke improves step by step. Now, you are in the process of recovery.

運動機能の評価:
基本的な評価として、中枢（脳、脊髄）からのコントロールの障害、すなわち麻痺や協調性などの障害の有無、関節の構造的異常の有無、疼痛や異常感覚の有無、関節可動域や筋力の測定を行う。
その結果をふまえて、より複雑で応用的な動作、つまり上肢全体の運動などを評価し、それらの問題が日常生活動作などにどう影響するかを評価する。

Clinical training : Assessment

Maki assesses the hand function of Mr. Kuroda using STEF.

Maki : This is a test to evaluate hand function. Firstly, please align the center of your body with the center of the board, and adopt a good posture. Secondly, please put your hand in the middle of the board on this side before the test. Thirdly, in the test, you will be asked to move items from one place to another quickly.

Kuroda : OK. Well, what is hand function?

Maki : Hand function includes grasp and pinch, finger extension, strength, coordination of joint movement, and other functions.

Kuroda : I see. You'll check it for me, right?

Maki : Yes, let's start. Test one is to move the ball from the right rectangle corner to the left same corner with your right hand.

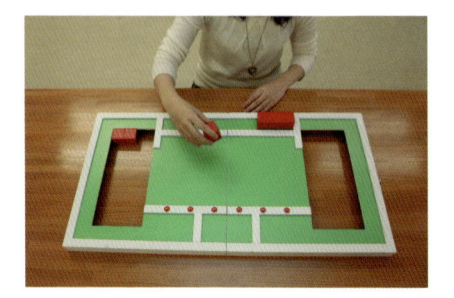

STEF:
(Simple Test for Evaluating hand Function)

上肢機能評価：
上肢の機能は、つかむ、握る、つまむ、ひっかける、すくう、押さえるなどの作用的な側面と、リーチ、移動、保つ、持つ、投げる、触る、コミュニケーションなどの目的的側面と、これらに関係する姿勢バランス、肩甲帯の安定と可動性、頭位と目と手の協調などを評価する。簡易上肢機能検査（STEF）、手指機能指数テスト（FQテスト）など多数の上肢機能検査から適切に選択して行う。

§4 *Physical functions*

Important consideration in assessment of physical functions

When OT students start the assessment of physical functions, there are some points to notice.

The highest priority is to avoid all risks and to prevent negative feelings, for example, anxiety, anger, and despair. Next, OT students may be puzzled about how to explain to patients how to make movement for the assessment. Many patients may not know any technical terms. So OT students need to think about what they should say instead of "abduct to the radial side of your thumb".

But a more difficult problem is how to have patients keep an appropriate position. They are not used to pain and paralysis, and so feel uneasy about movement. Some cannot understand OT students' instructions. In such cases, OT students need to be careful about trick motion. Most evaluation of physical functions requires specific posture and movement. OT students have two tasks. One is to master the method. The second is to devise how to have patients follow it correctly.

Question

What points do you need to think about for assessment of physical functions?

Clinical training : Assessment

> Hi! I am Taku. How are you?

> ……

TRACK 8

Section 5

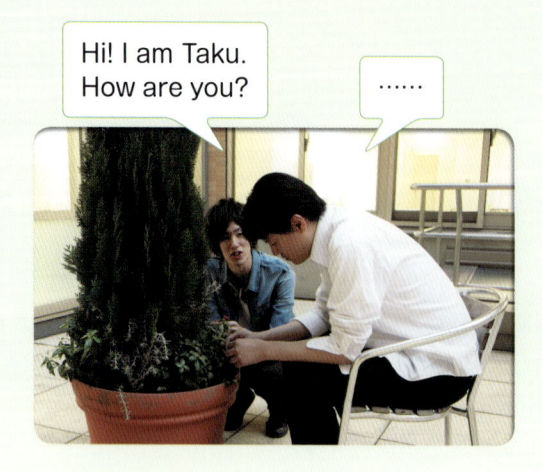

Psychological functions

Objective

Assess psychological functions

Now Taku is unusually nervous. He does not want to admit it, but he feels uneasy about assessing clients with mental disorders. He is worried about hurting the patients' feelings. He thinks that patients with mental disorders may be sensitive, and he has never met such people before. So he doesn't feel ready to carry out assessments.

§5 Psychological functions

SV : Taku, you seem a little discouraged.

Taku : I don't know what to do. I might hurt the patients' feelings. The patients are very sensitive, aren't they?

SV : Mm...well that's only partially true. Every person is sensitive and has a unique mentality. But some people have difficulties in their social relationships because of their personality or extreme moods.

Taku meets Mrs. Sada to assess using the Self-Rating Depression Scale. She is an outpatient.

Taku : Please look at the questionnaire. Could you read the questions and choose the most appropriate answer : never, sometimes, often, or always.

Sada : OK. *(after a while)* I've finished.

Taku : Thank you. Well, what do you like to do? Do you like handicrafts, games, walking, talking, reading, or something else? I'll do something with you.

Sada : Thank you. But how about next time? May I go home now?

Taku : Sure. Please take care and see you next week.

精神機能の評価:
重要なポイントとして、
①客観性
②再現性
③尺度の活用
などが挙げられる。
尺度としては、ライフイベントとストレス、うつ評価など、標準化された尺度がある。

Taku meets Mr. Takagi. He has some delusions and problems of thought and perception. He is occupied in farming as a part of an occupational therapy program.

Taku : Hello. My name is Taku. Nice to meet you.

Takagi : Hello. Do you see the stick over there? That is a signal flag to let me know something.

Taku : May I join you? I would like to do farming and talk with you.

Takagi : It doesn't sound good. I'm worried about the insects, so I change the weather. Does the stick mean something?

(Although it is a hot day, Mr. Takagi is dressed in a long-sleeved shirt.)

Taku : Are you cold?

Takagi : No. Atmospheric oxygen is dangerous for skin.

Taku leaves him

SV : Mm...as far as I saw, he was...he was not rejecting you. For the first meeting, you intervened enough with him. You've made a good start and we can go on from here.

Taku : OK, next time I will observe him to know how he is caring for himself and how he thinks about his interpersonal relationships.

§5 Psychological functions

What do you need to look at for assessment of psychological functions?

When you assess psychological functions, it is important to understand patients as a whole. OT students are apt to pay attention to the specific medical condition.

It is quite understandable that each positive or negative symptom attracts their attention. But they should evaluate not only the concrete content of delusions or hallucinations but all of the effects they have on patients' lives. If there are problems in the content and process of the ideas, how can OT students correct them?Depression is distressing, but it isn't easy to make improvements because it is an unconscious condition.

In addition, the state of physical functions is reflected in the mind. The influence of environment should not be neglected. What OT students should focus on are the effects that the mental disease has on self-expression, skills of living, and social participation. Through activities, everyone is related to and influenced by objects, people, and environment. Stress is caused by human relationships, sometimes leading to mental disorder.

Question

What do you need to look at for assessment of psychological functions?

Clinical training : Assessment

- Attention
- Integration of sensory information
- Executive functions
- Verbal communication
- Emotion Feelings
- Memory

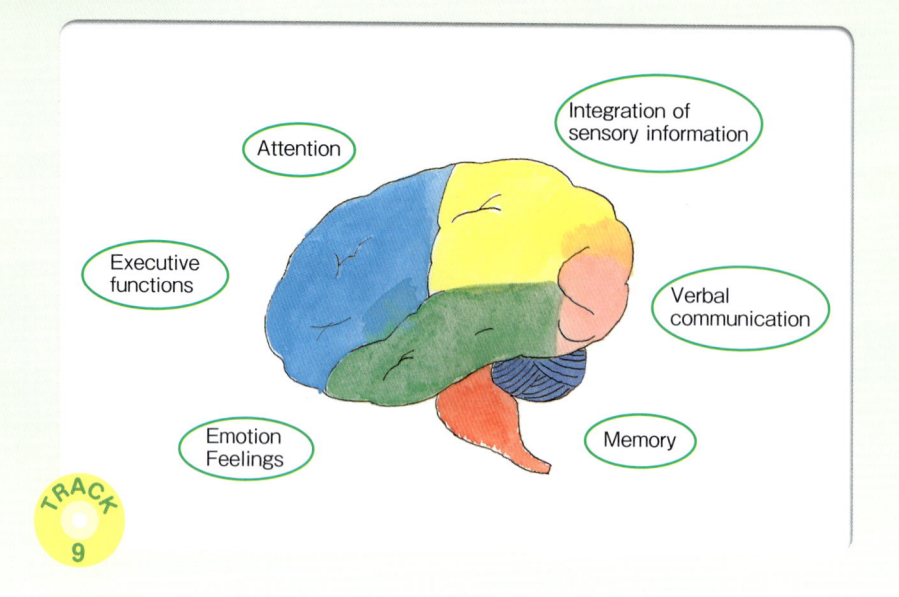

TRACK 9

Section 6
Higher brain dysfunction

Objective

To assess higher brain dysfunction

Maki is perplexed by a young patient, Mr.Nojima, who suffers from higher brain dysfunction. She is worried about how to assess his dysfunction. She cannot judge which is causing his problems, his dysfunction or his character. The more she thinks about it, the more puzzled she gets.

§6 Higher brain dysfunction

Maki : Well, let's talk about what you did this morning.
Nojima : Ah…I can't recall anything. *(laughing)*
Maki : Then, can you remember breakfast?
Nojima : *(He laughs more)* Maybe rice? I don't know. Please ask my mother.
Maki : That's OK. How did you come here?
Nojima : *(He laughs more and more)* Sorry.
Maki : Why are you laughing?
Nojima : I…I don't know why I'm laughing. I'm sorry. *(He stands up and sits down, moves his hand. He seems to be flustered)*
Maki : Please stay still.
Nojima's mother : He always laughs things off in this way. He can't do anything seriously.
Nojima : I'm so sorry. *(still laughing)*
Maki : OK. Let's try the next task. Do you remember how to start this personal computer? We've done it several times. If you don't remember, look at the notes you took last time.
Nojima : Notes? Did I? Really?

高次脳機能障害:
病気や事故などによる脳の部分的損傷が原因で起こる、注意・記憶・認知・言語・思考・学習・感情や行動の抑制などの障害である。
周囲の状況を理解し、それに合わせた行動をとることが困難になる。

Clinical training : Assessment

Maki : Yes you did. You usually carry a small notebook in your bag.
(He is staring at her)
　　　　Please take the notebook out, and check what to do.
Nojima : *(He is looking for the notebook)* I don't...what are you talking about?
Nojima's mother : Oh, I can't stand you.
　(She takes it out, hands it to him)
Nojima : *(He suddenly stands up)* Don't touch my things! *(He gets angry and starts crying)*
Maki : Take it easy. No one is touching your notebook. Please open it, and look for your notes about how to start the computer. I hope you can use the computer at some time in the future.

At a later time
SV : How about Mr. Nojima's assessment?
Maki : I couldn't do anything. Far from finishing any tests, I couldn't even start one.
SV : Well, what you should do is assess what's happening now. His dysfunctions are already pretty obvious.

高次脳機能障害の評価は、評価のプロセスで症状や特徴をよく観察することが重要となる。

§6 *Higher brain dysfunction*

Changes in the treatment of higher brain dysfunction

In the past, higher brain dysfunction meant, for example, aphasia, agnosia, and apraxia, constructional disability, disorientation, and spatial neglect. In those days, other cognitive problems were known, but not understood as the target of rehabilitation services.

In 2001, the higher brain dysfunction support model was introduced and the Ministry of Health, Labour and Welfare established the definition of the dysfunction. After that higher brain dysfunction became defined as dysfunction of attention, memory, executive function, consciousness of disease, communication, social behavior, and physical actions.

Recently, many evaluation methods have been developed to assess higher brain dysfunction, and there are more ways to support the dysfunction.

One of the important roles of OT for the dysfunction is to establish what and how the patient can do meaningful activities. Therefore occupational therapists observe the processes of activities and behaviors of patients carefully.

Question

How do you assess higher brain dysfunction?

Chapter 3

Completion of assessment and treatment

> Then, let's start the conference. Is everyone here?

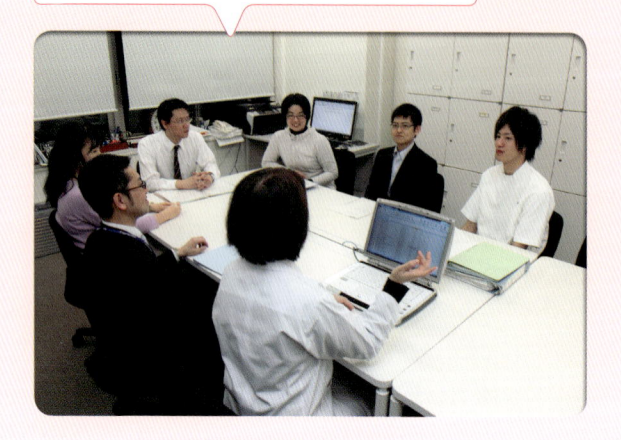

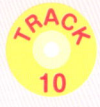

TRACK 10

Section 1

Conference for setting a goal and program in occupational therapy

Objective

Roles of conference participants

Taku is anxious about the assessment of Mr. Okada. He is supposed to prepare and set his rehabilitation goal before a conference. He reviews the results of several evaluations. But he loses his way of thinking about the client's problems and benefits.

§1 Conference for setting a goal and program in occupational therapy

SV : Taku, are you ready for the conference about Mr. Okada's case next Monday?

Taku : Actually, I haven't finished it yet. I don't know what all of his problems are.

SV : Well, did you assess him? What are the problems you found?

Taku : Well, I think I did enough. Mr. Okada has severe right hemi-paralysis, but this is on the way to recovery. I can help that. But if his right hand does not recover to a practically functional level, he will need to acquire skills to do everything he wants with his left hand instead of the right hand. His posture maintenance function is poor, so whether he stands or sits, his working efficiency and durability seriously decreases. He has depression. And sometimes he complains about difficulty in speaking.

SV : Right, em, but you haven't given an opinion there as an occupational therapist. One of the purposes of a conference is to gather the specialist opinion of each profession. What will other staff find interesting about your opinion?

---

conference:
症例検討会

利き手交換トレーニング:
Training for changing hand dominance

opinion as an occupational therapist:
作業療法士の独自の視点、理念とは専門性の基本である。それはクライエントにとって意味ある作業の可能化によるクライエントの生活や人生の再構築、役割の再獲得を実現することである。

Completion of assessment and treatment

Taku : Nothing....

SV : Mm...listen to other's opinions and review your ideas. And, you need to think about Mr. Okada's assessment from a different viewpoint. Have you asked him about his occupational needs and roles?

Taku : Yes, several times. But he only ever talks about returning to his previous job.

SV : What do you think his needs are?

Taku : I have no idea. He is a manager of a consumer electronics company. I cannot imagine his work or his daily activities in his office. And I do not know how much he will recover?

SV : Yes, he wants very much to be reintegrated into his family's life, doesn't he? Is that all?

Taku : Well....

SV : What can you do to help him to leave hospital?

Taku : Depending on his recovery, I will help him to get skills of activities of daily living (ADL) and instrumental activities of daily living (IADL), and abilities to return to office work. And I will try to know what he wants to do by himself.

---

occupational needs:
本人の意思だけでなく、例えば家族や職場、地域社会における当人への期待や役割、活用できる支援やサービスなどさまざまな要因により具体的なニーズが明らかになる。

occupational roles:
本人の生活や人生における役割を作業的側面からみた考え方。
人間関係や職業、成育歴や考え方などの背景が大きく影響する。

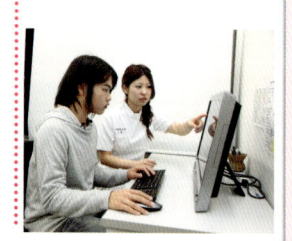

§1 *Conference for setting a goal and program in occupational therapy*

Conferences

In any medical or welfare facility, information gathering and opinion exchange are very important.

In the acute stage, the most important information is the results of medical diagnosis and treatment, and information about his or her context. Then, when the rehabilitation goal is being discussed, information about general welfare is important.

In other words, each participant in a conference has his/her role in providing specific information and opinions. Have you ever thought about the specific viewpoint of OT? What kind of evaluation is distinctive and provides specific information?

There are other important manners you should not forget. For example, you must be punctual and make remarks simply and clearly. In many cases, participants are very busy. Time is limited and needs to be used effectively. And you should not be too negative or too positive.

Question

What are the specific types of evaluation used in OT?

Chapter 3

Completion of assessment and treatment

Once I recover…

TRACK 11

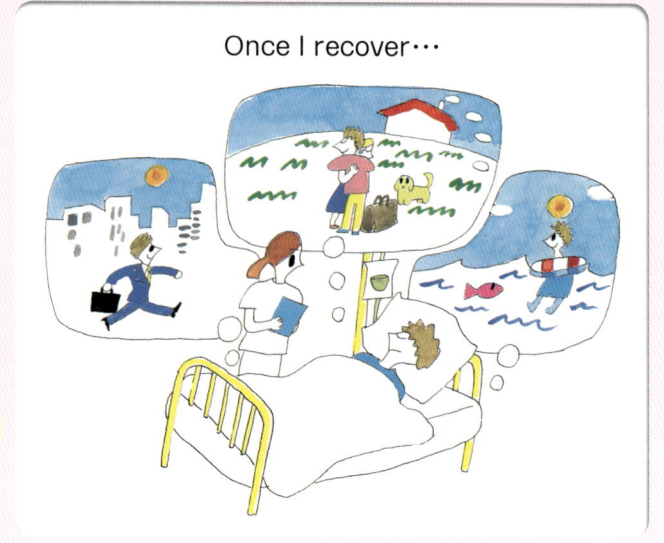

Section 2

Occupational therapy for physical dysfunction

Objective

What should OTs do for persons with physical disabilities?

Maki is building up her clinical experience. She has been trying various types of therapy she learned under instruction or supervision. She heard and saw a lot. She records everything she notices and discusses it with her supervisor often.

But she does not seem to understand everything.

§2 Occupational therapy for physical dysfunction

9:00 am. The clients enter the OT room one after another. Mrs. Wada who has suffered a stroke comes in.

Maki : Good morning. Can you move yourself from the wheelchair (W/C) to the exercise bed?

Wada : Yes, can you help me?

Maki : Sure.

She helped her to transfer from the W/C to the bed.

Please lie down. Firstly, I'll move your arms and legs. After that you try to turn over. If you can, get up and keep sitting on your own.

Wada : OK.

Mrs. Ogawa is suffering from rheumatoid arthritis.

Maki : How are you feeling this morning?

Ogawa : My hands have been stiff for a few hours, but my condition is better today.

Maki : Good. Let's try strength training and practice the way to protect your joints, after taking a paraffin bath with your hands.

Ogawa : I see. I would like to do some handicrafts like other patients. I like it.

Maki : The purpose of doing handicrafts for you is to maintain muscular power and range of motion of the joints by moving them actively. I will think about it for next time.

W/C (wheelchair):
車いす

ROMex (Range of motion exercise):
関節可動域訓練

RAのOT:
朝のこわばり、疼痛、関節の変形、易疲労、心理的影響などに配慮すれば、指から上肢全体を無理なく動かせる手工芸は機能維持だけでなく、趣味としても役立つ。

ハンドセラピーとOT:
外傷または手術により、手の関節や筋、末梢神経、皮膚などを損傷した場合、手や指の切断後の縫合や腱の再建などの場合のリハビリテーションをOTが担当する。

Chapter 3

Completion of assessment and treatment

Mr. Kishino whose two hands have severe burns.

Maki : Hello. How is your pain?

Kishino : It's OK, thank you. But are you torturing me now? I'm joking. I understand you're moving my fingers and hands to restore them even a little.

Ms. Nemoto is suffering from ataxia with dysmetria, asynergia and tremor.

Maki : What do you feel is inconvenient for you now?

Nemoto : That would be meals. I always spill stuff and it's so irritating.

Maki : OK. At supper time, I will come to your room and show you a better way to eat. Possibly, it might be useful to change your tableware, to use the elastick bandage or weight belt.

Nemoto : I want to exercise with wood pieces. It is very difficult to move my arm as I want. But I do feel like it's getting better gradually.

Mrs. Sada has damaged her spinal cord at level C6.

Sada : Listen! I could put on my socks! That small loop you sewed on the socks for me for use with a stick and hook is very useful! Thank you.

Maki : Not at all. I'm glad to hear that.

失調：
運動は常に多くの筋が協調して複雑な運動を可能にしている。それが障害され、筋力の調整や運動の方向や強さをコントロールできなくなるのが失調である。扱う道具の重さや形状を変える、筋に刺激を加えるなどの方法で対処する。

自助具：
運動機能的には不可能な動作でも、工夫を加えた道具(＝自助具)で可能にできることがある(078頁参照)。

§2 *Occupational therapy for physical dysfunction*

What is the real goal of OT for physical disability?

There is a question that almost all occupational therapists have been asked.

"Will I recover fully?"

This is a difficult question to answer. There are some clients who might fully recover but many of them will not. Indeed, occupational therapy cannot restore their physical functions completely, but occupational therapists may be able to help clients recover as they want. Everyone is constantly choosing a number of occupations which they need or want to do. Human life is defined by occupations.

It is important that better physical function facilitates possibilities and increases clients' chances of getting their life back.

There are three key points in OT with regard to physical disability. First, control of pain. Second, maximum maintenance of residual function. Third, if it is possible, to help recovery and establish goals for the client.

Question

How do you find the client's goal?

Chapter 3

Completion of assessment and treatment

TRACK 12

Section 3

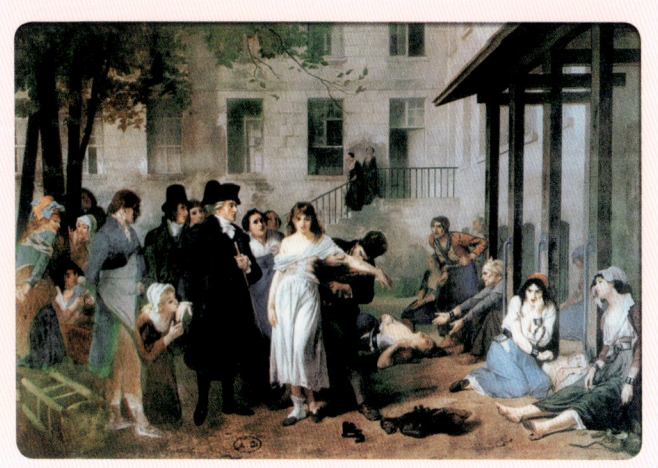

Occupational therapy for mental disorders

Objective

What should OT do for people with mental disorders?

Taku is at a loss in clinical training in the psychiatry department. He does not know which occupation is appropriate for which symptoms. In other words, he must think about purpose and adjustment for each occupation. And he is puzzled about how that connects to clients.

§3 Occupational therapy for mental disorders

SV : Mr. Takagi suffers from schizophrenia. You do some garden work with him, don't you? What do you think?

Taku : I talked with him a little. He is not a lazy man. He said he has some special relationships with celebrities, politicians, the staff of this hospital, and so on. And he had delusions about money.

SV : OK. How about thinking of some activities for evaluation and cure?

Taku : Woodwork? Weaving?

SV : You're not sure, are you? Em...try woodwork. Check his cognitive functions, for example, planning, understanding, concentration, endurance and how his symptoms change under different stresses.

Mr. Takagi and Taku are in the OT room.

Taku : Today, I'd like you to make a shelf from wood. First, please write a plan and confirm the procedure and the materials.

Takagi : *(silence)*

Taku : OK, I'll help you. First of all, let's decide the size.

Takagi : It's up to you to decide.

Taku : No. It is important that you decide everything. I can just help you.

Takagi : Shut up! You're good-for-nothing!

Schizophrenia
(統合失調症)：
陽性症状：
幻覚・妄想・焦燥感・興奮・攻撃的・奇異な行動や服装・空笑・場にそぐわない感情・思考の障害。
陰性症状：
自閉・引きこもり・無為・情動の平板化・情動鈍磨・思考の貧困・意欲や発動性の欠如・仕事などが長続きしない・快感消失・非社交性・注意の低下。

＊冒頭の絵画は、トニー・ロベール・フルーリによる"ピネルが精神病患者を解放する図"である。

Completion of assessment and treatment

Mr. Takagi has gone back to his room.

SV : Taku, what do you know about Mrs. Shirai?

Taku : She does garden work too. She suffers from bipolar disorder. Now she is shifting to a manic state. In the manic state, she tends to cause trouble in interpersonal relationships.

SV : Why?

Taku : At the last conference, it was confirmed that if her need for identification, sense of belonging and sympathy is not met, she shows egocentric behavior. So she cannot establish relationships with others.

SV : Actually, she and her family hope she can leave hospital and play the role of housewife and mother. Before the next conference about her case, we should assess the functions necessary to fulfill that role.

Taku : What functions do we assess?

SV : Not we but you. Check if she can handle various household chores. But the most important point you need to be careful about is, in a hospital it is not easy to evaluate what kinds of dissatisfaction or uneasiness she feels at home.

社会性の回復:
精神的な障害やハンディキャップを抱えるクライエントの社会性の回復は非常に重要な目標となる。歴史的に長期の社会的入院や自宅での軟禁状態、無為好褥や引きこもりなどの状態が非常に多かった。

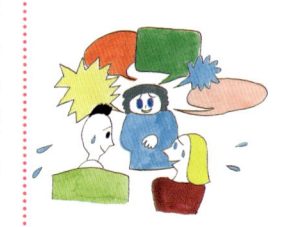

§3 *Occupational therapy for mental disorders*

OT for unseen disabilities

It is quite normal if someone feels incompatibility with people with mental disorders.

Throughout history, many such people were feared and excluded by society.

Why? Because people don't easily understand what they rarely see, and overreact when they see someone different from them. People pay too much attention to symptoms, but not enough to their background.

One of the objectives of OT for mental disorders is to clarify the relationship between a symptom and its background. What kind of feelings are influencing people's attitudes? What kind of conditions cause stress? What is the meaning of occupation? What are their potential functions of living, studying, working, and playing.

Question

What do you feel about people with mental disorders?

Completion of assessment and treatment

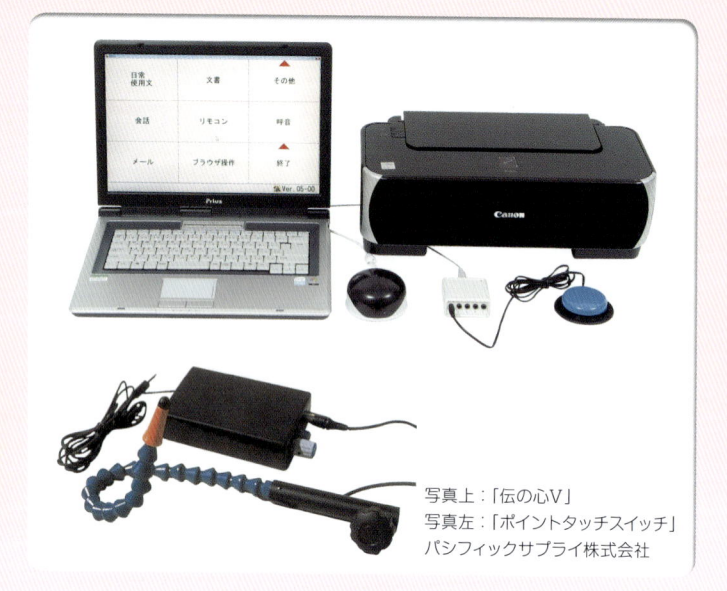

写真上:「伝の心V」
写真左:「ポイントタッチスイッチ」
パシフィックサプライ株式会社

Section 4

Occupational therapy for developmental disabilities

Objective

What can OT do in school?

Maki gets an opportunity for full-day training at a special support school. She meets a girl named Kumiko with physical disabilities and difficulty in speaking. So even when she has a desire to urinate, she cannot ask for someone's help. She also has problems with dressing because of her physical disabilities. SV instructs Maki to tackle the problem.

§4 Occupational therapy for developmental disabilities

SV : Kumiko is a smart girl, but it is difficult for her to speak.

Maki : She needs some devices to make sounds instead of her voice.

SV : Good. But how can she operate the device? She has severe cerebral palsy. She cannot move her arms and legs well.

Maki : I think I can make switches which she can push. It's easy to push something when it's fixed to the desk or floor, or so on.

SV : Does she always have to carry the switch throughout the day?

Maki : No. But is there any pattern about the times when she needs to use the bathroom? She cannot eat and drink freely. If she drinks water at a set time, it might be predictable when she'll need the bathroom.

SV : Yes, the teacher has already recorded her activity every day.

Maki : I'll confirm her bathroom times from the record. Then I'll assess her physical function to check if she can use the switches.

SV : Yes, you should talk with her teacher and the speech therapist.

Completion of assessment and treatment

After assessment, Maki tries the switch with Kumiko.

Maki : Look at this switch. If you want to go to the lavatory, please push the switch. Then you can make a sound to ask for someone.

Kumiko tries to push the switch. She can.

Maki : Good. If you like, push it again please.

Kumiko pushes again.

Maki : Thank you. Next is about how to put on and take off clothes easily in the lavatory? May I add changes to your clothes so that I can help easily? If you say yes, push the switch. Nothing? OK. If you say no, push the switch. OK. You don't want to make changes to your clothes.

Teacher : Kumiko likes fashion, so maybe she's afraid of you making strange, unbecoming, or plain functional clothes.

Kumiko pushes the switch again with a laugh.

Maki : I see. Well, if you happen to like the clothes I make, please try them.

Teacher : What is the benefit of the switch other then calling someone? Kumiko gets irritated in a variety of situations where she cannot communicate with others...when it's not possible to do as she hopes or desires.

Maki : It's worth thinking about that together. Of course with Kumiko too.

§4 Occupational therapy for developmental disabilities

The new field of OT for developmental disorders

Until recently, OT for developmental disorders was provided in hospitals, facilities for special disorders and partially in schools for special education.

In recent years, advances in medical treatment and the promotion of employment for people with disabilities have expanded the opportunities for people with developmental disorders to participate in society.

As a result of this trend, the role of occupational therapy is expected to increase, too. For example, in schools for special needs education, OTs increasingly work collaboratively with teachers, and it is possible to participate in education services as an external specialist.

Question

What can OT do for people with developmental disorders?

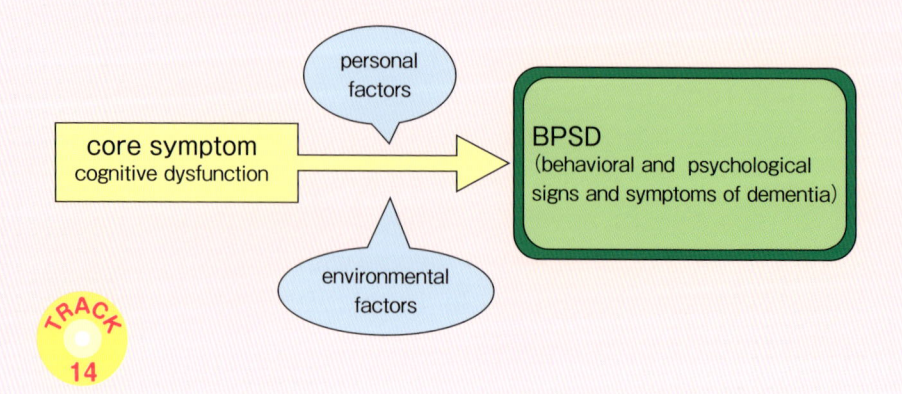

Chapter 3 Completion of assessment and treatment

```
core symptom          →    BPSD
cognitive dysfunction      (behavioral and psychological
                            signs and symptoms of dementia)
```
personal factors
environmental factors

TRACK 14

Section 5 Occupational therapy for elderly people

Objective

What should OT do for elderly people?

Taku is in clinical training at a special elderly nursing home. He thinks the objectives of OT for elderly people are to treat them kindly and to maintain their function. He knows about dementia, because his grandfather suffered from it. He thinks that it is impossible to treat dementia, and that one must simply endure it. But he notices at once that he was wrong.

§5 Occupational therapy for elderly people

Taku has to plan and do group therapy for persons who are feeling uneasy when walking.

SV : Care staff may be too busy to walk here with them. Let's go and see. It's a good opportunity to observe how they usually spend their time.

Taku : *(to a woman)* Hello. How about walking to group therapy with me?

(While walking)

Participant : But I like gate ball more.

Taku : I'm sorry, but gate ball is on Tuesdays.

At group training

Taku : Hello everyone. How are you? To begin with, let's stretch our bodies.

(after 10 minutes)

Next, I'm going to give you a small quiz about the Showa era. Let's make groups of three people and discuss the answers in your group.

(after 15 minutes)

Let's take a small break. After the break, we're going to play big balloon.

Participant : This is too much. Let me go back to my room.

After group training

SV : It's good to help them talk about the Showa era. Recalling old times is useful to form a sense of belonging.

高齢者の作業療法：
高齢者の作業療法の主な目的は、機能の改善、維持による介護予防である。主には趣味や娯楽的な活動やグループ体操、過去の回想や歌唱、異世代との交流などを通じて、身体機能や精神機能のみならず、社会性が保たれるように働きかける。

Chapter 3 — Completion of assessment and treatment

Taku is in the OT room. Some clients want to reduce their pain with a hot pack, some do handicrafts as they like.

Kaise : I couldn't sleep well last night. My back and my knees hurt. I think your massage will be effective.

Taku : I'm sorry, but we haven't learned massage techniques yet.

Kaise : Oh well, please try anyway.

Taku does the massage as requested

Care worker : May I talk to you? Some clients need a special spoon for their meals. Can you do an evaluation and prepare the spoon?

Taku : OK, I can evaluate them tomorrow.

Care worker : Thank you.

A few people are wandering in the corridor. One of them, Mr. Kubo, comes into the OT-room.

Kubo : Where is my house? Is this my house?

Care worker : *(to Taku)* When he was young, he used to go home to take a nap in his lunch hour. *(to Kubo)* Have you finished lunch? How about going home with me?

Taku : I see. There is a reason for each act of care.

Tobe : *(embroidering)* A needle and thread, please.

Taku : Coming up!

認知症高齢者の問題行動：
中核症状は残念ながら改善しないことが多い。しかしそこに環境の要因が加わって起こる問題行動などは予防、改善することが可能である。日々の観察やケアに関わるスタッフの情報交換によって、手掛かりがつかめることが多い。

§5 Occupational therapy for elderly people

OT for elderly people

Recently, the importance of the preventive approach has increased in long-term care.

Main concerns are maintaining physical function and how we approach dementia. In the past, the approach for the well-elderly was poor, but now we understand that a preventive approach needs to begin from middle age.

We can divide the symptoms of dementia into two groups. One is core symptoms: that includes cognitive disorders such as memory disturbance, impaired orientation, disorder of ideas and judgment, ataxia, and agnosia. The other group comprises behavioral and psychological signs and symptoms of dementia: BPSD. BPSD includes anxiety, fretting, delusions, illusions, depression, roaming, hyperactivity, dirty behavior, railing, violence, resistance, and collection. OTs must focus on both of these aspects.

Question

What is the difference in OT between the two types of symptoms of dementia?

Chapter 3

Completion of assessment and treatment

It is so hard to live with disabilities in the community.

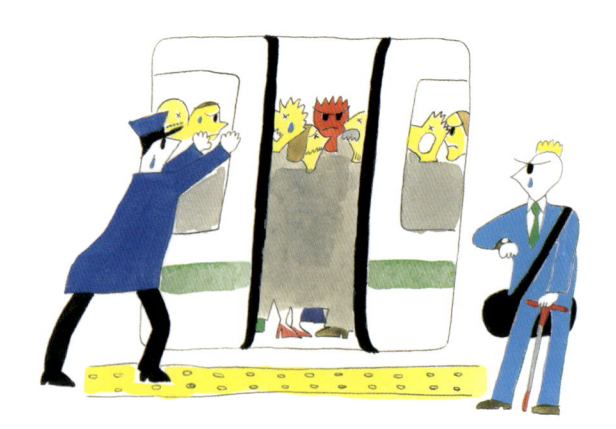

TRACK 15

Section 6

Community-based occupational therapy

Objective

How can CBR be implemented in Japan?

Maki has known some students with disabilities who were absent from class regularly because they were receiving rehabilitation services. Maki is wondering whether environmental barriers, including the place rehabilitation services are provided, prevent people with disabilities from full participation in society.

§6 Community-based occupational therapy

Maki is in a rehabilitation center. An occupational therapist guides her.

Therapist: This is the rehabilitation room.

Maki: Can anyone use it?

Therapist: No. Children with developmental disabilities and clients covered by care insurance can't use it. But they can use other facilities.

Maki: If a client wanted further recovery, where should they go?

Therapist: That's difficult to answer. It depends on the meaning of recovery. There are various kinds of clients. Some want to make a full recovery and get back to their lives as they were, and some want functional recovery training for returning to their job, and some come here for interpersonal relationships.

Maki: What training do they do here?

Therapist: Mostly, it's continuation of training from a previous hospital. If necessary, the program can be changed according to client's demand. Recently, needs concerning re-starting work have increased.

Maki: OT for work?

介護保険サービス:
65歳以上の人で日常生活に支援が必要になったときに利用できる。
さらに加入年齢の40歳から65歳まででも、以下の特定疾患の場合は介護保険サービスを利用できる。
がん・関節リウマチ
筋萎縮性側索硬化症・後縦靭帯骨化症・骨折を伴う骨粗鬆症
初老期における認知症・進行性核上性麻痺、大脳皮質基底核変性症およびパーキンソン病・脊髄小脳変性症・脊柱管狭窄症・多系統萎縮症
糖尿病性神経障害、糖尿病性腎症および糖尿病性網膜症
脳血管疾患・閉塞性動脈硬化症・慢性閉塞性肺疾患
両側の膝関節または股関節に著しい変形を伴う変形性関節症

059

Chapter 3
Completion of assessment and treatment

Therapist : Oh yes, for example, before they start looking for work, they want to recover their function so that they can stick it out.

(They enter next room)

Next is the life-long education service room.

Maki : What is the purpose of this room?

Therapist : Well, education expands a person's possibilities. And that's also true for people with disabilities. There are skills relating to computers, hobbies, sports and so on.

(They enter the dining room)

Next is the dining room and the shop managed by people with disabilities. This is social participation and training too.

Maki : That's great.

Therapist : Cleaning of the facilities and reception work has been entrusted to them, too. I think if it's possible here, it's possible in the community, too. What do you think the next step should be?

Maki : I think we should tell the community about that, and change ordinary people's way of thinking.

CBR
(Community Based Rehabilitation)：
CBRの定義（2004年 WHO、ILO、UNESCO、UNICEFの合同報告書）障害のあるすべての子供と大人のためのリハビリテーション、機会の均等、ソーシャルインクルージョンのための総合的な地域開発の中の一つの戦略であり、障害のある人や、その家族、地域住民、教育、職業および社会サービスの協力を通じて実行される。

CBRの目標：
1. 障害者が身体的、精神的能力を最大限発揮でき、通常のサービスと機会を利用でき、地域や社会において積極的な貢献者となるよう促進すること。
2. 参加の障壁を取り除くといった、地域社会での変化を通して障害者の人権を促進、保護するよう地域社会を活性化すること。
CBR研究会 <http://www.cbr.in/book/jointpaper2005.html>

§6 Community-based occupational therapy

Institution-based rehabilitation (IBR) versus community-based rehabilitation (CBR)

Physical exercise machines, assistive technologies, and professional therapists may be available in IBR because there are big rehabilitation institutions in cities. However, there is little equipment and a few specialized personnel for rehabilitation in the countryside and in developing countries.

The healthcare policy of the Japanese government places emphasis on establishing a system of community care. Rehabilitation services such as OT, PT, and ST are also covered by the long-term care insurance system. In CBR, therapists work with individuals with disabilities on modification of environments, and on education for care givers.

In 2004, the ILO, UNESCO, and WHO published a joint position paper. CBR was defined as follows. CBR is a strategy within general community development for the rehabilitation, equalization of opportunities and social inclusion of all people with disabilities. CBR is implemented through the combined efforts of people with disabilities themselves, their families, organizations and communities, and the relevant governmental and non-governmental health, education, vocational, social and other services.

Question

What do you think about CBR in Japan?

Chapter 4

Client-centered occupational therapy ⟨Mr. Okada's case : CVA⟩

```
                    Health condition
                           │
          ┌────────────────┼────────────────┐
          ↓                ↓                ↓
    Body functions  ←→  Activity   ←→   Participation
    Body structures
          │                │                │
          │                ↓                │
          │         ┌──────┴──────┐         │
          ↓         ↓             ↓         ↓
              Environmental    Personal factors
                factors
```

TRACK 16

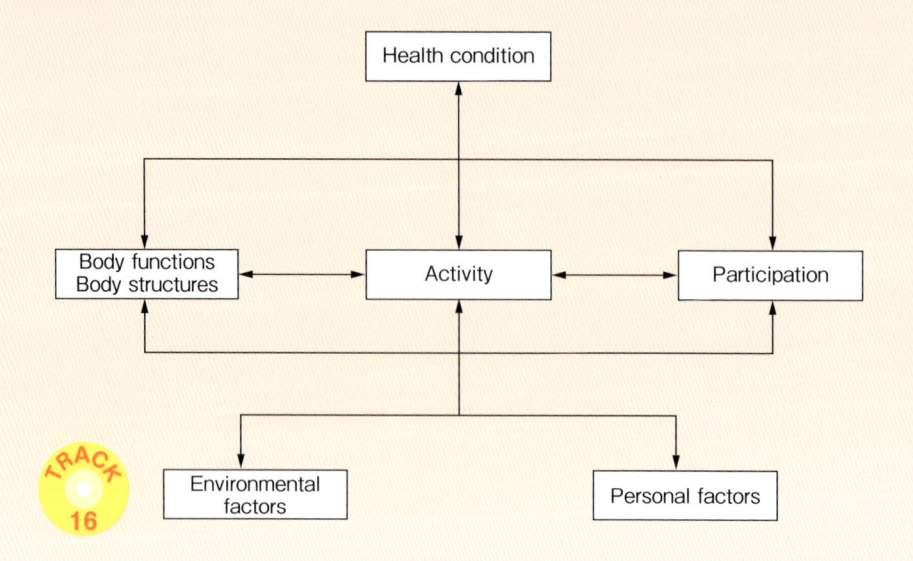

Section 1

ICF : International Classification of Functioning, Disability and Health

Objective

What ICF can establish about clients?

Taku works hard to identify Mr. Okada's occupational problems and what he should do for him. He can list some disabilities, but he cannot grasp the essential part of Mr. Okada's problems and needs. He is confused about each particular factor, so he loses their connection to each other.

§1 ICF:International Classification of Functioning, Disability and Health

SV : Taku, are you ready to start Mr. Okada's program?

Taku : Honestly speaking, I don't have much confidence about the priority of his problems.

SV : OK. Show me your work.

Taku : OK. He has severe right hemi-paralysis. According to the Brunnstrom stage, his right upper arm and fingers are stage 3, and his right leg is stage 4. He can do part of the voluntary moves from the synergy pattern. He has sensory disorder and limitation of range of motion. His posture is asymmetric. He can sit stably for a long time...

SV : Did you read the comprehensive implementation plan for rehabilitation? I think you have identified each factor in his problems, but you haven't found out the relationships among them. You should look again at Mr. Okada's case based on ICF.

Taku : I'm sorry, I don't know about ICF. Is it only for classification?

SV : No, you haven't understood it. Classification is only the first step. The second step is identification of problems and discovery of relationships between them. These steps are very useful and interesting. Try it.

ICF参照図書
「国際生活機能分類——国際障害分類改定版」世界保健機関 障害者福祉研究会。中央法規出版、東京、2003

Chapter 4

Client-centered occupational therapy 〈Mr.Okada's case : CVA〉

After assessment on ICF

Taku : I went through Mr. Okada's case again with ICF. I'm surprised because it helped me to think about him from different points of view.

SV : For example?

Taku : Well, the problems I identified were only physical matters. I was focusing on whether he could go back to work. I didn't notice what factors were relevant to his need.

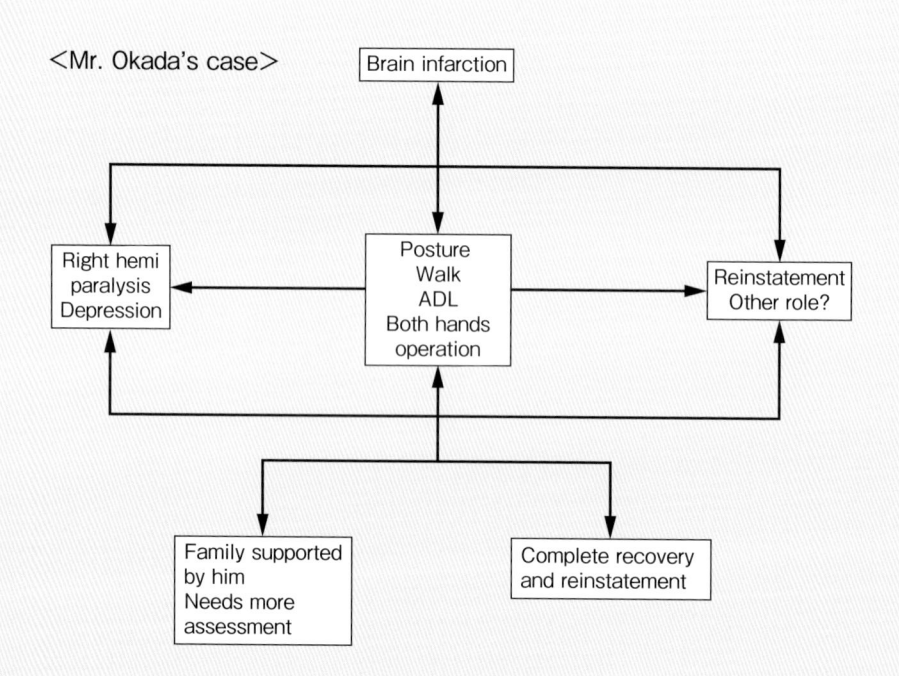

<Mr. Okada's case>

```
                    ┌─────────────────┐
                    │ Brain infarction│
                    └────────▲────────┘
                             │
    ┌──────────────┐   ┌─────┴──────┐   ┌──────────────┐
    │ Right hemi   │   │  Posture   │   │ Reinstatement│
    │ paralysis    │◄──│  Walk      │──►│ Other role?  │
    │ Depression   │   │  ADL       │   │              │
    └──────▲───────┘   │ Both hands │   └──────────────┘
           │           │ operation  │
           │           └─────▲──────┘
           │                 │
    ┌──────┴────────┐   ┌────┴──────────────┐
    │Family supported│   │Complete recovery  │
    │by him          │   │and reinstatement  │
    │Needs more      │   │                   │
    │assessment      │   │                   │
    └────────────────┘   └───────────────────┘
```

§1 ICF:International Classification of Functioning, Disability and Health

Practical use of ICF

ICF is not merely a tool for classification of human function related to health. When we want to describe a person's physical function and state of disorder, ICF is useful as a framework to organize information.

We know that there are strong relationships between human function, activity and participation. In addition, environmental factors and personal factors play a role. Usually, it is not easy to notice these relationships. For example, when we have functional impairments, we pay attention only to the improvement of the function.

Unfortunately, in many cases, it is difficult to recover completely, but giving up, we should look at the overall state of health using ICF.

Question

What is the role of ICF in OT?

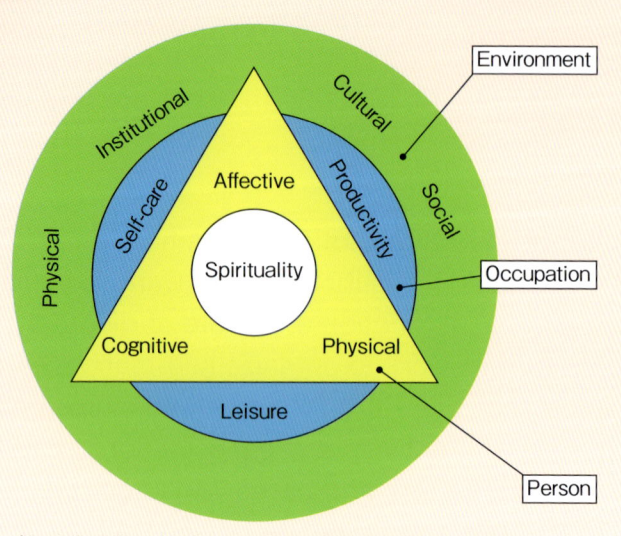

Chapter 4 — Client-centered occupational therapy ⟨Mr. Okada's case : CVA⟩

(Enabling Occupation: An Occupational Therapy Perspective, Canadian Association of Occupational Therapists, 1997)

Section 2 — A practice based on CMOP (Canadian Model of Occupational Performance)

Objective

Clients know about their needs

Taku interviews Mr. Okada using COPM. He has a strong desire to recover physically. Taku tries to focus on daily activities rather than physical functioning. However, he does not explain his real intention and uneasiness.

§2 A practice based on CMOP (Canadian Model of Occupational Performance)

Taku: I would like to know your occupational issues because I'm an occupational therapist. I'll ask you some questions using the Canadian Occupational Performance Measure, which is also called COPM. Could you tell me the activities you want to do, need to do, and are expected to do?

Okada: I want to walk.

Taku: I see. Where do you want to walk?

Okada: Anywhere. I can go anywhere if I can walk.

Taku: I see what you want to say. But shall we start at the smaller step such as going to the bathroom or going to the dining room?

Okada: I want to go to the bathroom by myself.

Taku: All right. Going to the bathroom is one of your problems now. Is there anything else? What do you have to do?

Okada: I need to go back to work.

Taku: What kind of job do you do?

Okada: Deskwork.

Taku: Do you use a computer?

Okada: Yes.

カナダ作業遂行モデル（CMOP）：
1997年にEnabling Occupation（CAOT, 1997）で発表され、Enabling Occupation II（CAOT, 2007）で改訂された。

カナダ作業遂行測定（COPM）：
1990年に初版が発表され、2005年に第4版が出版されている。

クライエント中心の実践：
カナダ作業療法士協会（CAOT）は1980年からOTとは何かを議論し、クライエント中心の実践こそがOTの本質であるとした。ここでのクライエント中心とは、クライエントと作業療法士とのパートナーシップを基本とする。クライエント中心は米国表記ではclient-centeredだが、CAOTの定義を生かすためにclient-centredと英国表記されることもある。

Chapter 4 Client-centered occupational therapy 〈Mr.Okada's case : CVA〉

Taku continues the assessment.

Taku : Next, you have to think about how important those activities are for you on a scale from one to ten. Ten means extremely important. One means not important at all. How important is going to the bathroom for you?

Okada : Em...eight.

Taku : Right, so going to the bathroom is quite important for you.

Okada : Yes.

Mr. Okada rates the importance of each occupational issue.

Taku : Next, can I ask you to rate the way you do this activity now? How well can you go to the bathroom? Ten means you do it very well. One means you can't do it at all.

Okada : Em...five.

Taku : OK. Your performance is in the middle. How about your satisfaction? You should say 10 if you are satisfied your current performance about going to the bathroom. You should say 1 if you aren't satisfied at all.

Okada : I'll say 7 because I can get help in the hospital. I don't have to do it independently here.

Mr. Okada rates performance and satisfaction scores on each occupational issue.

Taku : OK, thank you for your cooperation. We will work on these kinds of things in our occupational therapy.

COPM:
この評価法は、①作業の特定、②重要度の評定、③遂行度と満足度の評定、④遂行度と満足度の再評価という4段階で行われる。初回評価では①から③までを行う。OTはクライエントが自分の作業の問題を考えやすいように、1日の流れを話してもらったり、以前の仕事や趣味を聞いたり、将来の希望を聞いたりする。評定には、1から10までの数字が書いてあるimportanceとperformanceとsatisfactionの3枚のカードを使う。(Mary Lawほか著, 吉川ひろみ訳. COPMカナダ作業遂行測定 第4版, 大学教育出版, 2006)

§2 A practice based on CMOP (Canadian Model of Occupational Performance)

A first step towards client-centered practice

It is very important to realize client-centered practice. How can we do it? Firstly, therapists should know the client's perspective. Client-centered practice is based on the idea that the person who has the most information resources about the client is the client themselves.

One of the assessment tools to know the client's perspective is the Canadian Occupational Performance Measure (COPM). COPM is based on the Canadian Model of Occupational Performance (CMOP).

Person, environment, and occupation are factors in CMOP. Physical (doing), cognitive (thinking), and affective (feeling) are components of the person. Cultural, social, physical, and institutional are elements of the environment. Self-care, productivity, and leisure are areas of occupation. Spirituality is essence of self.

CMOP was developed by the Canadian Association of Occupational Therapists in 1997 and revised to the Canadian Model of Occupational Performance and Engagement (CMOP-E) in 2007. Occupational engagement is a broader concept than occupational performance.

Question

What is the focus in CMOP?

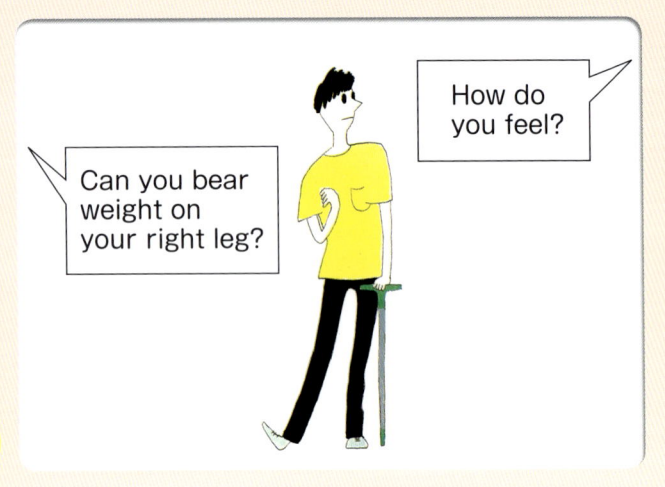

Chapter 4 Client-centered occupational therapy 〈Mr.Okada's case : CVA〉

> How do you feel?

> Can you bear weight on your right leg?

TRACK 18

Section 3 Clinical reasoning to think in action

Objective

To explain your clinical reasoning

Taku finally starts Mr. Okada's training. SV asks him what he is doing and why? Taku can explain what he is doing, however, he cannot explain why he is doing it. Because he had no idea about Mr. Okada's occupational therapy, he copied a plan for a person with hemi-paralysis from his textbook.

§3 Clinical reasoning to think in action

Taku : I will facilitate voluntary movement because Mr. Okada's paralysis is severe.

SV : That's one type of clinical reasoning, called procedural reasoning. You should think about other types of reasoning. His functional abilities, environment, and personal factors should be considered when you plan his occupational therapy program.

Taku : Ah…I didn't give it enough thought.

Taku meets Mr. Okada in the OT room.

Taku : We'll try to use a computer today because you said you need to use a computer in your job.

Okada : My right hand needs to be recovered for using a computer.

Taku : Well, you can use your left hand. When you try to sit straight, using a computer will have a positive influence on your recovery.

Okada : I'm sitting straight.

Taku : Well, maybe not as straight as you think. *(Taku brings a mirror.)* See… your posture is leaning over.

Okada : You're right. …I'm tired. Can I finish for today?

Taku : Yes. Are you OK?

Okada : I'm just a little tired.

行動の理由：
臨床で行われている行動には理由がある。この検査でこの結果が出たからこの診断で間違いない、というように臨床での行動を理由づけていくことをクリニカルリーズニングという。1990年代初めにアメリカの文化人類学者Cheryl Mattinglyの協力を得てOTのクリニカルリーズニング研究が行われた。研究者はOTと患者のやりとりをビデオに撮り、ビデオを見ながらOTに、なぜその行動をとったのか理由を聞いた。その結果、OTでは評価結果から介入を決めるといった手続き的（procedural）リーズニング以外のリーズニングが多く使われていることが明らかになった。

Chapter 4 *Client-centered occupational therapy 〈Mr. Okada's case : CVA〉*

Taku : Mr. Okada seems upset.

SV : Yes, well, you didn't respond to the way he's feeling. He wants to be able to exercise. And when you showed him his posture in the mirror, he felt that he was very far from recovery. You should think about what's happened in his life story. That's narrative reasoning.

Taku : How can I do it?

SV : Well, think about what you did. You'll be able to think in action as you develop as an occupational therapist. Theory guides practice. Practice is explained by theory. Therapists need to think in acting, and act with thinking. That's a reflective practitioner.

Taku : I see I am far from being a reflective practitioner.

SV : Well, it's a life-long learning process.

クリニカルリーズニングのタイプ：

OTのリーズニングとして、手続き的(procedural)、叙述的(narrative)、相互交流的(interactive)、条件的あるいは状況的(conditional)、実際的(pragmatic)、倫理的(ethical)リーズニングがあるとされている。

考えてから行動(think then action)するのではなく、自分の行動の理由を考えたり(think on action)、行動しながら考える(think in action)ことで、プロフェッショナルとして成長できるといわれている。行動を振り返ることを省察(reflection)といい、反省的実践家(reflective practitioner)になることが推奨されている。

吉川ひろみ. 作業療法士としての成長の仕方. OTジャーナル, 39 (4), 280-284, 2005

§3 *Clinical reasoning to think in action*

Types of clinical reasoning in OT practice

Clinical reasoning is the thought process that guides practice. Research on the clinical reasoning of expert therapists reveals that they use different types of reasoning and switch from one type to another very fluently (Mattingly, 1991).

Procedural reasoning involves thinking how to go forward in therapeutic process. Procedural reasoning is similar to identifying diagnosis from symptoms revealed by evaluation. Students learn procedural reasoning in class.

Narrative reasoning involves understanding the client's story through listening and observing. The client's subjective experience is the focus of narrative reasoning.

Interactive reasoning involves the relationship between therapist and client. Interactive reasoning cannot be learned in class. In occupational therapy programs, when the client and therapist do things together, the experience becomes a part of the client's life story.

Conditional, pragmatic, and ethical reasoning are also used in OT. Therapists choose the appropriate type of reasoning for each situation and switch from one type to another. Although students and beginner therapists have to stop to think what type of reasoning they should use, expert therapists can act fluently and effectively.

Mattingly C. What is clinical reasoning? American Journal of Occupational Therapy, 45 (11), 979-986, 1991

Question

What is clinical reasoning for OT?

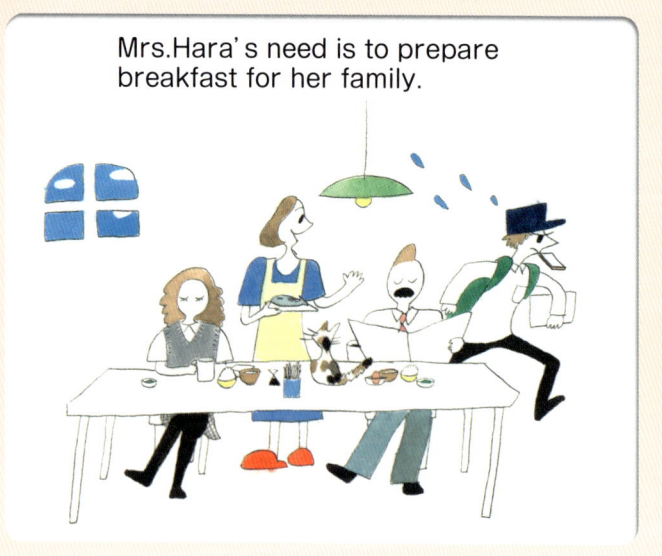

Chapter 4 Client-centered occupational therapy 〈Mrs.Hara's case : RA〉

Mrs.Hara's need is to prepare breakfast for her family.

TRACK 19

Section 4

A practice based on MOHO (Model of Human Occupation)

Objective

How to practice MOHO

Maki thinks it is necessary to arrive at some consensus about the meaning of domestic work for Mrs. Hara. Mrs. Hara hopes to make her family comfortable by herself. Maki would like to respect her will, but does not think Mrs. Hara ought to do everything herself to show her devotion to her family.

In addition, Maki has to know what domestic tasks are most important for her and her family. SV suggests an intervention based on MOHO.

§4 A practice based on MOHO (Model of Human Occupation)

Maki : I'm reluctant to do practice based on the Model of Human Occupation (MOHO). In fact, I don't know about MOHO very well.

SV : Check the reference books. MOHO has been used with a wide variety of clients.

Maki and SV refer to MOHO

Maki : MOHO focuses on motivation for occupation, maintaining positive involvement in the roles and routines, skilled performance of necessary life tasks, and the influence of physical and social environment.

SV : There are many assessment tools in MOHO such as the Interest Checklist and the Role Checklist, the Occupational Questionnaire (OQ), and the Occupational Self Assessment (OSA). Those are self-report style evaluations.

Maki : The Assessment of Communication and Interaction Skills (ACIS), the Assessment of Motor and Process Skills (AMPS) are used by means of observation. The Occupational Circumstances Assessment : Interview and Rating Scale (OCAIRS) and the Occupational Performance History Interview-II (OPHI-II) are interviews.

SV : The Model of Human Occupation Screening Tool (MOHOST) is developed for gathering information about the effect of volition, habituation, skills, and environment on clients' occupational participation. MOHOST is implemented by means of observation, interview, and chart review.

MOHO：人間作業モデル
Gary Kielhofnerは1980年にAmerican Journal of Occupational Therapyに人間作業モデル（MOHO）を発表し、1985年に初版を出版した。2007年には第4版が出版され、第3版までは邦訳「人間作業モデル」（山田孝他訳）が出版されている。
MOHOウェブサイト〈http://www.moho.uic.edu/〉
このモデルは意志（volition）、習慣化（habituation）、遂行能力（performance capacity）という3要素から構成される。意志には、個人的原因帰属（personal causation）、価値（value）、興味（interest）が含まれる。習慣化には習慣（habit）と役割（role）が含まれる。環境には物理的（physical）環境と社会的（social）環境があり、意志、習慣、遂行能力に影響を与えるものとして概念化されている。

Maki : I think it is important to identify the essential parts of Mrs. Hara's volition. She's too obsessive about keeping house by herself for her family. But I think that others could do it just as well. The result would be the same. So I think that she and I should confirm her functions, daily activities for her family, role, and environment.

SV : Good. What will you do next?

Maki : I would like to hear from her family about their views on her role. I think it's important that her and her family's view about her role at home is compatible with her disease.

After assessment

Maki : I think you want to be a good homemaker and make your family's life comfortable, don't you?

Hara : Yes, of course.

Maki : But you need to be aware of your condition. For example, let's think about breakfast. You want to make breakfast for your family, even though your hands are usually stiff every morning.

Hara : I miss making breakfast for them. I want to give them a good start everyday.

Maki : I know. Your children say they've enjoyed your special breakfast every morning from childhood, but they say they are not happy to see you're having a hard time cooking. I think you need some changes with regard to your family.

Hara : What kind of changes?

Maki : One might be to stop cooking in the morning. You can prepare for the next day's breakfast when you cook dinner. And you should ask for help from your family. The most important thing is that you feel happy in the morning.

MOHOの実践例：
ハラさんは、家族のために家事をしたいという意志は強いが、力仕事ができないという遂行能力の問題がある。関節にかかる負担を減らすために、やり方を変えたり、自助具を使ったりすることは、ハラさんの習慣を変えることになる。家族に家事を頼むことは、ハラさんの価値観とは合わないし、家族の態度（社会的環境）も影響する。今までのように家事を行えないことで、ハラさんの役割も変わっていく。このようにMOHOを使うことでクライエントの状態を理解することができる。

ハラさんは、家族に家事を負担させないということに価値を置いている。またハラさんは、マキが提案する病気への対処法についても興味を示している。ハラさんの価値観は、家事も病気への対処も、できるだけ自分でなんとか行いたいということなのかもしれない。病気など人生の危機に対して、自分はここまではできるだろうというある程度の自信（個人的原因帰属）があるはずだ。

§4 A practice based on MOHO (Model of Human Occupation)

Importance of knowing background of occupation

In the Model of Human Occupation (MOHO), humans are conceptualized as made up of three interrelated components. These are volition, habituation and performance capacity.

Volition means the need or desire to act, with three sub components. These are personal causation, value (what's important and meaningful to do?) and interests (what's enjoyable and satisfying to do?).

Habituation means the process of habits and roles influencing behavior in familiar environments and situations.

Performance capacity to do occupation depends on several factors. These include physical bodily systems and mental or cognitive abilities, such as memory and planning. In addition performance capacity and environment influence each other.

Occupational therapists must think about why the client wants to do a specific occupation, how the occupation is done in the client's daily habits, and what role is performed by doing the occupation.

Question

What do you think about human occupation?

Chapter 4 — *Client-centered occupational therapy 〈Mrs. Hara's case : RA〉*

Some useful equipment and devices

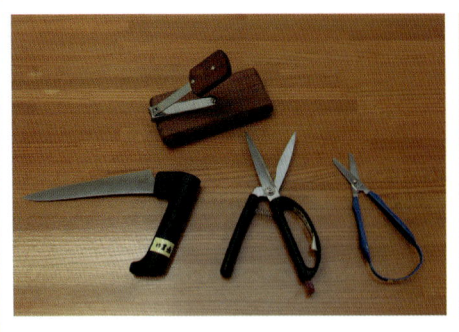

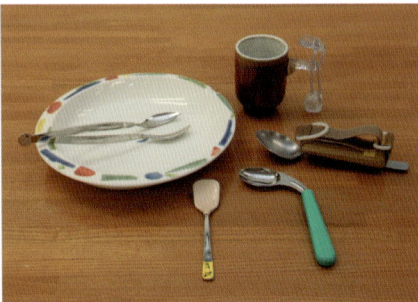

TRACK 20

Section 5 — Joint protection for ADL and IADL

Objective

How to live protecting joints

Maki is working on Mrs. Hara's case. She is suffering from rheumatoid arthritis, but she wants to keep house and do enjoyable things. But her wrists and finger joints are very weak, so Maki worries about protecting her joints.

§5 Joint protection for ADL and IADL

Maki: Well, to be honest, your wrist and finger joints are too weak and have some deformation, so for many things you will need to find new ways of doing them.

Hara: That sounds difficult. When I feel pain in my hands, I can't do anything in the ordinary way. Is that included in the treatment?

Maki: Yes, it is included. But I would like to tell you about precautions to prevent tiredness, pain, and deformation.

Hara: How?

Maki: There are these important points. They are joint protection, energy conservation and environmental modification. In other words, don't grasp and pinch strongly and, don't get tired…

Hara: Excuse me? Don't grasp strongly? I have to grasp many things strongly.

Maki: When and what do you want to grasp strongly?

Hara: When I do housework. For example, cleaning, washing, ironing, making meals and so on.

Maki: Can you ask for your family's help.

リウマチの関節保護：
リウマチでは痛みへの配慮や関節保護が非常に重要である。
まず痛みやこわばりの出現の傾向や、関節の変形、運動機能を評価する。
次に日常生活動作の中で問題となる作業を明らかにし、方法や道具を工夫し、負担を軽減し、これまでどおりに作業を遂行できるように本人、家族と検討する。

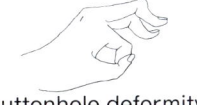

buttonhole deformity

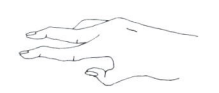

swanneck deformity

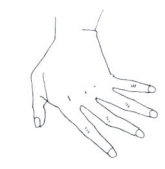

ulnar driff deformity

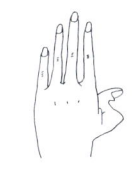

Z shape deformity

079

4 Client-centered occupational therapy ⟨Mrs.Hara's case : RA⟩

Hara : But my husband and children work hard, so I'd like to make a comfortable home for them by myself.

Maki : Well, I'll give you general points to pay attention to. After that, we have to talk about how you can do what you want.

Hara : I see.

Maki : The first thing is about pain and deformation of joints. You must think about when your pain increases. You should avoid ill-use of joints. For example, grasping something firmly, holding objects which are too heavy.

Hara : So...I need to pay special attention when I cook.

Maki : And you mustn't keep the same posture for a long time. For example, when you move your hand, you had better put your arm or elbow on the table. Because your joint will become stiff.

Hara : If I don't actually try these things, I don't understand.

Maki : OK. We'll try it together. And then you should avoid getting tired and keep strength and range of motion in your joints.

Hara : OK, I'll try to do what you tell me.

§5 Joint protection for ADL and IADL

Life with rheumatoid arthritis

Rheumatoid arthritis is a debilitating disease. Its characteristic is progressive decline of physical strength and function.

There are three quick rules to prevent this. The first is the protection of joints. The second is conservation of energy. The third is adjustment of environment. The purpose of these rules is to avoid pain, tiredness, and transformation of joints.

But there is another point that is as important as implementing these rules. That is consideration of the quality of life of each client. Quality of life depends on how one lives everyday. So occupational therapists must always keep focus on activities of daily living. By following the three rules, clients can avoid damage to their quality of life. The difficulty of occupational therapy for rheumatoid arthritis lies in approaching the two aspects together, prevention of progression and improvement of quality of life.

Question

What are the important things in OT for people with rheumatoid arthritis?

Chapter 4

Client-centered occupational therapy ⟨Mrs.Hara's case : RA⟩

A kitchen plan which Maki made for Mrs.Hara.

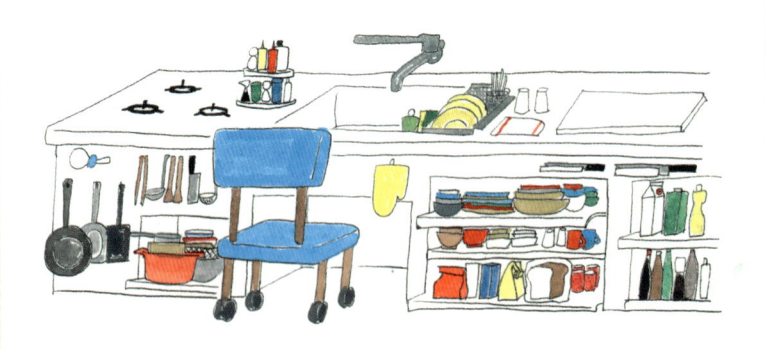

TRACK 21

Section 6

Environmental modification

Objective

How to use devices and modify the environment

Maki visits Mrs. Hara's house to evaluate and modify her environment. As expected, her house and her living environment are typical and, in suffering from rheumatism, she experiences various difficulties in her daily life.

§6 Environmental modification

Maki : Firstly, I'd like to see your kitchen. You want to prepare breakfast every morning, don't you?
Hara : Yes, I do. Here is my kitchen.
Maki : What are the problems?
Hara : I become tired after standing for a long time to cook, and I have to move around because the storage spaces are dispersed here and there.
Maki : Which storage spaces in particular can't you use easily?
Hara : The ones close to the floor or the ceiling. They are too low or too high.
Maki : You should avoid kneeling down or standing on tiptoe, because the load rests upon the foot. Let's take out the stored items, and move them to easier places to use. I will do it and you give me directions.
Hara : Thank you.
Maki : Next, I would like to see cooking tools, and tableware.
Hara : Here you are.
Maki : The one-handled pan is a load on the wrist, so use a two-handled pan.

ハラさんのキッチンプランで重要な点は、
①関節保護
②疲労防止
である。
マキのプランの利点は、
・調理台が平ら
・椅子に座って調理できる
・収納位置が低い
・水道のレバーへの配慮
などである。
欠点は、
・重い鍋やビンを持ち上げないといけない
・まな板に遠すぎて無理な姿勢になる
などである。

人―環境―作業の関係：
OTでは、人（person）、環境（environment）、作業（occupation）の関係（P-E-O）を考える。ハラさんがうまく料理が行えるかどうかは、人（ハラさんの心身機能）と環境（台所や道具）と作業（料理の種類）が相互に関連し合った結果である。

Chapter 4 Client-centered occupational therapy 〈Mrs.Hara's case : RA〉

Maki : I recommend placing a chair or stool in front of the sink, and making a space where your legs can fit under the sink. In that way you can cook sitting on a chair.

Hara : That's a good idea. It's possible to cook without getting tired.

Maki : Next, do you mind changing some tools and equipment? For example, water taps, some tools for cooking, and so on. If you change to special tools or equipment which are easy to grasp, then you'll have less load on your joints.

Hara : Well, that's expensive and my joints are still strong.

Maki : I see. But the earlier the stage of rheumatoid arthritis that you start at, the more effective the results will be. Next, I want to see the bathroom. And may I observe the way you take a bath, getting into the bath?

Hara : Do I have to take my clothes off?

Maki : No. I just want to see your movement.

Hara : By adjusting my living environment, can I prevent progress of my disease?

Maki : Yes, but as well as that, let's practice exercises for rheumatoid arthritis.

障害予防:
疾病予防と同様に障害が重度化することを予防することができる。OTは、進行性の疾患や、二次的な障害の発生が予測される場合に、環境を調整したり、効果的な作業の仕方を指導したりすることにより、予防的な関わりができる。

毎日の身体的負担は少なくても継続的に負担が蓄積することで起こる障害がある。手根管症候群などはcumulative trauma disorders:CTD (蓄積外傷疾患) という。

§6 Environmental modification

Interaction between persons, environments, and occupations

Occupational performance results from the dynamic relationship between a person, environment, and occupation. The figure illustrates interactions. Three components (person, environment, occupation) interact continually across time and space. The closer they overlap, the more harmoniously they are interacting.

Environmental modification and choosing appropriate occupations allows increasing occupational performance.

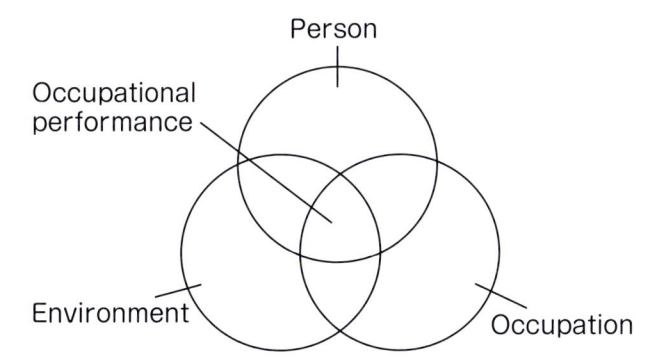

Law M et al. The person-environment-occupation model: A transactive approach to occupational performance. Canadian Journal of Occupational Therapy, 63 (1), 9-23, 1996

Question

How do you modify environments?

Chapter 5

Fundamental concepts

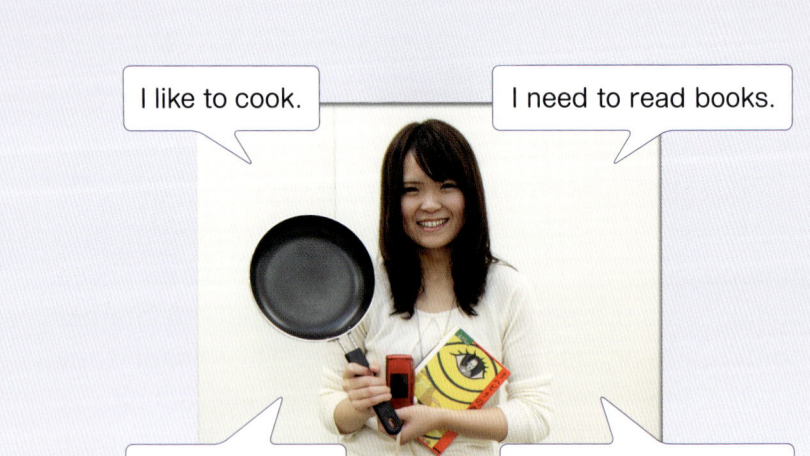

I like to cook.

I need to read books.

I love to talk with friends.

I am an occupational therapy student.

TRACK 22

Section 1
Occupation

Objective

To understand yourself as an occupational being

People like doing particular things, occupations. Meaningful occupations bring enjoyment and fulfillment and help to establish a person's identity. People are defined by their occupations. Every person is an occupational being.

§1 Occupation

Maki: I have to study. I have to do my part time job. I'm very busy.
Taku: Do you have any time for hobbies?
Maki: I used to like playing piano.
Taku: Wow. You're a pianist.
Maki: No. I'm not a pianist. I haven't played piano for a long time. I don't have a piano. How about you? Do you have any hobbies?
Taku: My hobbies are fishing, and shopping, and playing tennis, and cooking…
Maki: You have many occupations.
Taku: Yes. I learned patience through fishing. Shopping is always exciting for me. Playing tennis keeps me fit. Cooking for others maintains and expands my social network. I am what I do.
Maki: You're a very occupational being.

OTの人間観:
今の自分は、今までの自分がどんな作業をしてきたかで決まり、将来の自分はこれからどんな作業をするかで決まる。このような人間観は、doing、being、becomingと表現される。
昔は、どの地域の誰の子として生まれるか、男か女か、障害があるかないかによって、何をして一生を過ごすかが、ほぼ決まっていた。これはbeingによってdoingが決まるということである。しかし、人は誰でもかけがえのない個人として尊重されるべきだという、人権意識の高まりにより、居住地や職業の選択ができるようになってきた。Doingはoccupationのもっとも簡単な表現である。自分が何をするか、しないかで、今の自分 (being) のあり様が決まり、将来の自分 (becoming) もつくられていくのである。
英語の勉強を一生懸命すれば、世界の人々と一緒に働くようになり、グローバルな人になれる。

Definitions of occupation

1. Chunks of culturally and personally meaningful activity in which humans engage that can be named in the lexicon of the culture (Clark et al, 1991).

2. Groups of activities and tasks of everyday of life, named, organized, and given value and meaning by individuals and a culture. Occupation is everything people do to occupy themselves, including looking after themselves (self-care), enjoying life (leisure) and contributing to the social and economic fabric of their communities (productivity) (CAOT, 1997).

3. An activity or set of activities that is performed with some consistency and regularity, that brings structure and is given value and meaning by individuals and a culture (Townsend & Polatajko, 2007).

4. The things people do everyday as individuals, in families and with communities to occupy time and bring meaning and purpose to life (ISOS, 2007).

1．作業とは、文化的個人的に意味をもつ活動の一群で、文化の語彙の中で名づけられ、人間が行うことである。

2．作業とは、日々生活で行われ、名づけられている一群の活動や課題で、個人と文化によりその価値と意味が付与されたものをいう。作業とは、自分の身の回りのことを自分で行うセルフケア、生活を楽しむレジャー、社会的活動、経済的活動に貢献する生産活動など、人が行うすべての営みのことである。

3．一貫性や規則のある遂行の活動のセットで、構造をもち、個人や文化により価値と意味が与えられたもの。

4．家族やコミュニティの中で人生に意味と目的をもたらし時間を使って、人が個人として日々行うこと。

§1 Occupation

What is occupational science?

Occupational science was founded by occupational therapists in the late 1980s to generate knowledge about human occupation. It studies the things that people do in their everyday lives and how those occupations influence and are influenced by health and well-being. Important concerns within occupational science are how, when, where, and why people determine their occupations.

The World Federation of Occupational Therapists (WFOT) recognizes that knowledge of human occupation is the essential foundation of occupational therapy and provides a theoretical framework for occupational therapy research.

WFOT recognizes that concepts from occupational science enable occupational therapists to understand their client's subjective experiences and unique perspectives (WFOT, 2010).

Activity

Please introduce yourself as an occupational being

Fundamental concepts

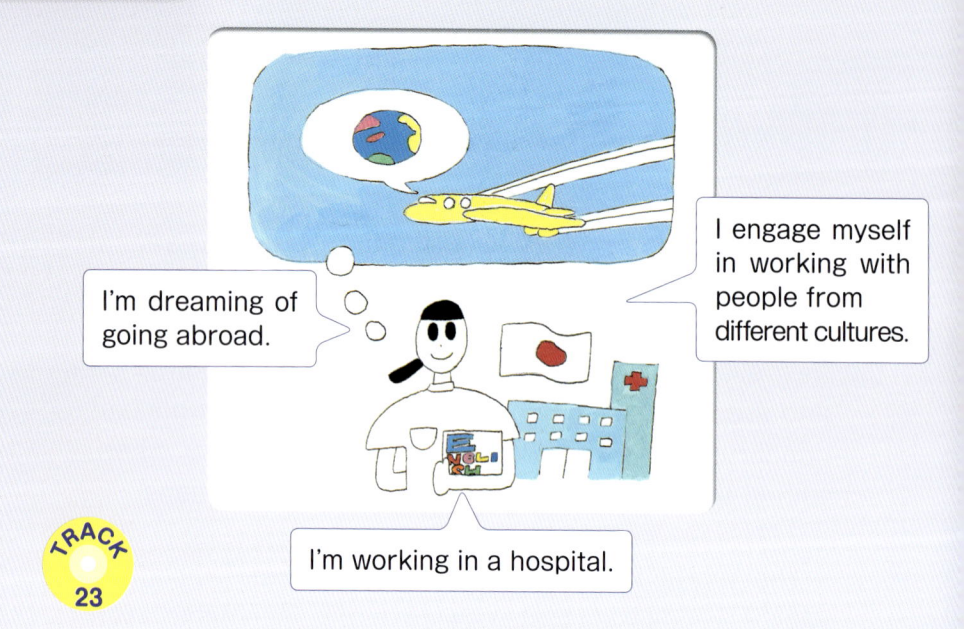

I'm dreaming of going abroad.

I engage myself in working with people from different cultures.

I'm working in a hospital.

TRACK 23

Section 2

Engagement in occupation

Objective

To distinguish between occupational engagement and occupational performance

Occupational engagement is involvement for being, becoming, and belonging, as well as for performing or doing occupations (Wilcock, 2006).
Occupational engagement is not only doing by one's self but also feeling and/or thinking about occupations.

§2　Engagement in occupation

Taku : A friend of mine got engaged recently. It's making me think about my future.
Maki : Do you have any plans to get engaged?
Taku : No plans! How about you?
Maki : I want to go abroad.
Taku : Oh really? When will you go abroad?
Maki : Well…after I graduate, I'll work at a hospital and do community service for several years. Then I'll apply to overseas volunteer programs. Occupational therapists can make people engage in meaningful occupations throughout the world.
Taku : Ah…so that's why you're studying English so hard!
Maki : English alone is not enough. But English is the most useful language for communication because the greater number of people speak English as a second language. Communication between non-native speakers can be easier than with native speakers. In addition, occupational therapists focus on occupations that include non-verbal communication.
Taku : I want to engage in an occupation meeting a nice girl!

国際基準をもつOT：
国境を越えて働くOTは比較的多い。世界作業療法士連盟（WFOT）はOT資格を得るための教育基準を定めており、WFOTが認可したOT養成校を卒業すれば、世界中の多くの国や地域でOTとして働くことができる。多様性に満ちた世界の国や地域では、OTの役割は非常に広い。ストリートチルドレンの健康的な成長を支援したり、内戦後の地域復興のために働くOTもいる（Kronenbergほか、2005）。WFOTは国際的に活動するOTのための情報と資源の共有を目的としたウェブサイトOTION（Occupational Therapy International Outreach Network、オーシャンと読む）を立ち上げた。

Fundamental concepts

Occupational...

Performance: The result of a dynamic, interwoven relationship between person, environment, and occupation over a person's lifespan. Performance requires the ability to choose and satisfactorily perform meaningful occupations (Townsend & Polatajko, 2007).

Development: The gradual change in occupational behavior over time, resulting from the growth and maturation of the individual in interaction with the environment. There are three levels of development: micro, meso, and macro (Davis & Polatajko, 2010).

Identity: How an individual sees the self in terms of various occupational roles. An image of the kind of life desired (Kielhofner et al, 2001).

Potential: People's capacity to do what is required and what they have the opportunity to do, to become the people they have the potential to be (Wicks, 2005).

作業に関連する概念:

作業遂行は、カナダ作業療法士協会(CAOT)がカナダ作業遂行モデルの中で説明した。

作業発達のミクロレベルとは作業を習得していくプロセスであり、メゾレベルとは個人の発達であり、マクロレベルとは人類の発達を指す。

作業アイデンティティは、人間作業モデルの評価法OPHI-Ⅱの開発の中で概念化された。

作業ポテンシャルは、オーストラリアの作業療法士、アリソン・ウィックスが高齢女性へのインタビューを通して命名した概念である。

§2 Engagement in occupation

Rick engages in marathons without running

Rick was born in 1962 to Dick and Judy Hoyt. As a result of oxygen deprivation to Rick's brain at the time of his birth, Rick was diagnosed as a spastic quadriplegic with cerebral palsy.

Though Rick could not walk or speak, he was quite astute and his eyes would follow people as they moved around the room.

In 1972, a group of engineers at Tufts University built Rick an interactive computer. When the computer was first brought home, Rick surprised everyone with his first words on the computer. "Go, Bruins!" The Boston Bruins were in the Stanley Cup finals that season. It was clear from that moment on that Rick loved sports.

In the spring of 1977, Rick told his father that he wanted to participate in a 5-mile benefit run for a lacrosse player who had been paralyzed in an accident. Although not a long-distance runner, Dick agreed to push Rick in his wheelchair. They finished the 5 mile run. That night, Rick told his father, "Dad, when I'm 'running', it feels like I'm not handicapped."

Together, Dick and Rick have completed 1,000 races, including marathons and triathlons (6 of them being Ironman competitions). In 1992, they biked and ran across the U. S. completing 3,735 miles in 45 days.

Team Hoyt<http://www.teamhoyt.com/>

Question

Give an example of occupational engagement

Fundamental concepts

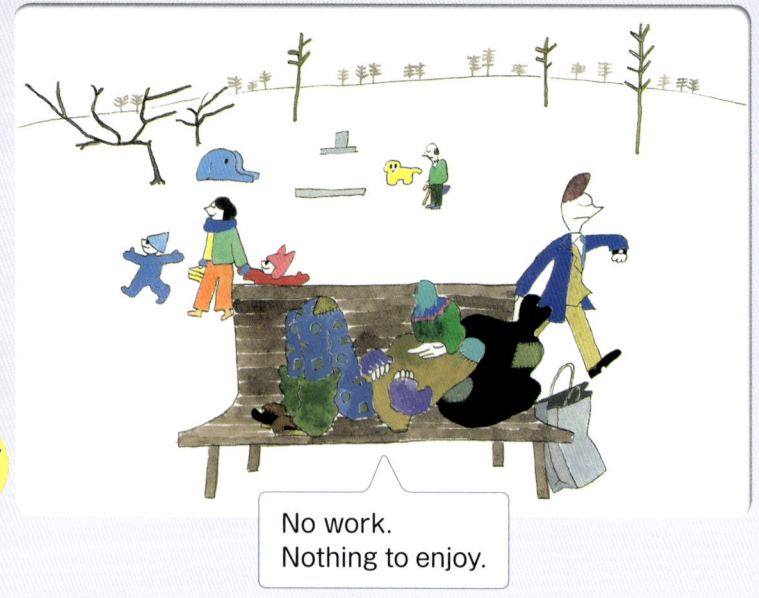

No work.
Nothing to enjoy.

Section 3
Occupational justice

Objective

To identify situations of occupational injustice

Whilst social justice addresses the social relations and social conditions of life, occupational justice addresses what people do in their relationships and conditions for living (Wilcock&Townsend, 2000).

It is occupationally unjust if people do not have opportunity for access to meaningful occupations within their community.

§3 Occupational justice

Maki : I read a book about poverty and homelessness.

Taku : Somebody suggested I get a license such as a therapist's license because my parents were afraid of me becoming a freeter*1 or a NEET*2.

Maki : Children who are abandoned by their parents can't get enough education. So they have to do low-paying jobs. Economic recessions hit them directly. They can't pay rent. Life as a homeless person makes it more difficult to find a job.

Taku : Do occupational therapists work with such people?

Maki : Yes, we do. There are people who don't have a home, job, money and food, not only because of the economic recession but also because of the early discharge policy in psychiatric hospitals. Occupational therapists support them to reconstruct their lives.

Taku : Wow, that seems very difficult.

Maki : It would be easier if society accepted diversity and supported different lifestyles.

*1 permanent part-timer
*2 Not in Employment, Education or Training

職業に就くことは大事な作業:
フリーター（freeter）は日本語、ニート（NEET）は教育も職業訓練も受けていない若者を指す英国の造語。日本では、働く意欲がないことを意味して使われることがある。どの社会においても仕事は成人の重要な作業である。カナダのエリザベス・タウンゼントが述べた作業療法士の社会的理想（social vision）と、オーストラリアのアン・ウィルコックの作業は人間の基本ニードだとする考えが合流して、作業的公正（occupational justice）という概念が生まれた。Justiceは正義あるいは公正と訳されている。ある事柄間の関係が丁度よい（just）かどうかが問われる。Injusticeは理不尽な差別や不平等な状態を指す。

Terms associated with occupational injustice

Occupational deprivation: A state of prolonged preclusion from engagement in occupations of necessity and/or meaning due to factors which stand outside of the control of the individual (Whiteford, 2000).

Occupational alienation: The outcome when people experience daily life as meaningless or purposeless (Stadnyk et al, 2010).

Occupational marginalization: It occurs when some social groups more than others are denied or restricted in making choices and decisions about their participation in everyday occupations, often resulting from invisible expectations, norms, and standards (Townsend & Wilcock, 2004).

Occupational imbalance: Allocation of time use for particular purposes (Stadnyk et al, 2010)

作業的公正と不公正:
作業的公正(occupational justice)が守られていない状態を作業的不公正(occupational injustice)という。作業剥奪、作業疎外、作業周縁化、作業不均衡は、作業的不公正の例である。

作業剥奪(occupational deprivation)は、当事者以外の理由で行う作業がない状態であり、謹慎など罰として与えられることがある。

作業疎外(occupational alienation)は、作業を行ってはいるものの、自分の作業とは感じられない状態である。

作業周縁化(occupational marginalization)は、会社の中で主要な仕事を与えられず、お茶くみなど瑣末な仕事しか行っていない状況を指す。

作業不均衡(occupational imbalance)は、行うべき作業が多すぎたり、逆に少なすぎたりする状態である。

§3 *Occupational justice*

Justice

Justice is generally accepted to be an ideal vision of society. American philosopher John Rawls (1971) emphasized individual rights, responsibilities and liberties. Procedural justice is to hear the view of all different groups of people. Restorative justice is the restoration of perpetrators of wrongdoing and restitution to victims. Distributive justice is proper distribution and redistribution of resources in society (Stadnyk, Townsend&Wilcock, 2010).

Occupational justice means protection of rights to engage in meaningful occupations.

Nobody wants to experience unfairness, be undervalued or not respected. Occupational justice means protection of rights to engage in meaningful occupations.

Boys not being allowed to learn ballet; girls being forced to do housework. These are examples of sex-role stereotyping that creates injustice. Geographic isolation, unemployment, and incarceration are more examples of occupational injustice. People with disabilities tend to experience occupational injustice because they cannot do what they need and want to do because of physical and social environmental factors (Whiteford, 2000, 2010).

Question

How is our society occupationally unjust?

Fundamental concepts

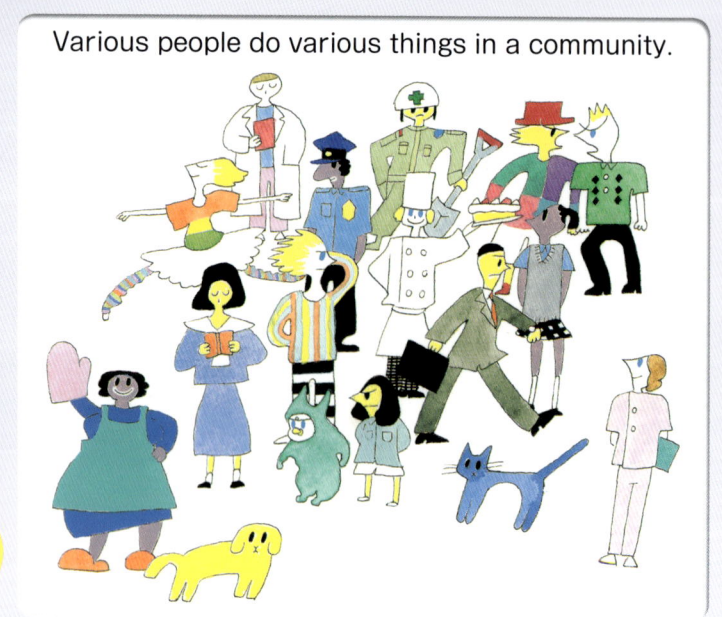

Various people do various things in a community.

TRACK 25

Section 4

Inclusion

Objective

To imagine an inclusive society

The inclusion of one thing in another involves making it a part of the second thing. Inclusion refers to the belief that all individuals should be able to participate fully in the activities of life with the same benefits and opportunities (WFOT, 2009).

§4 Inclusion

Taku : I visited a rehabilitation center yesterday. It was a big facility. It has a hospital, kindergarten, elementary and middle high schools, dormitories, and sheltered workshops.

Maki : Children with disabilities have to live apart from their parents to go to special schools. But more parents are working for educational integration. Educational integration means that children with disabilities learn with other children.

Taku : I have heard of community integration.

Maki : Community integration means people with disabilities live in the same community as all other people.

Taku : Integration sounds great.

Maki : Inclusion is better than integration. Inclusion is based on the idea that everyone is different. Society should be made up of people with different abilities. We shouldn't stigmatize people who have disabilities. We have to learn how to live together.

Taku : I guess if society includes people with disabilities, there's no need for integration.

Maki : You've got it.

インクルージョン：
障害児・者、少数民族、特定の階層の出身者などの少数派 (minority) が、その社会を構成する多数派 (majority) とは異なる地区に住み、異なる仕事をしている状態においては、多数派のコミュニティ (mainstream) に少数派を統合 (integration) する必要があった。
インクルージョンは、最初から、多様な人々が存在する状態を指す。ソーシャルインクルージョン (social inclusion) は、社会的包摂と訳されることもあり、1990年代以降日本でも普及しつつある考え方である。身体状態や人種や居住地などの違いを理由に排除 (exclusion) するのではなく、すべてを包み込むような社会 (inclusive society) の創造を目指す。

Fundamental concepts

In the past, our society was more exclusive and less flexible. People who had chronic disease or disabilities were hospitalized or institutionalized. People with impairments went to special schools then worked at sheltered workshops. Rehabilitation centers and sanatoriums were built in out-of-the-way places. Minority groups such as particular ethnic groups, people with disabilities, and gays and lesbians were excluded from mainstream society. The dominant groups in mainstream society were men, able-body adults, the rich and heterosexually oriented people.

Inclusion is based on the ideas of difference and the beliefs that every person is unique, has intrinsic dignity and has the right to make choices about life.

People shape and are shaped by their environment. Environment influences how people engage in occupations. An inclusive society supports people choosing and performing meaningful occupations.

インクルージョンは、すべての個人は同等の利益と機会をもち、日常の活動に完全に参加できるべきだという信念を示す言葉であり、インテグレーションに続いて登場してきた。

§4 Inclusion

The protection of human rights in society

Human rights are protected by society. The United Nations adopted the Universal Declaration of Human Rights in 1948.

"All human beings are born free and equal in dignity and rights (Article 1)" (United Nations, 1948)

Occupational therapy is the art and science of enabling engagement in everyday living, through occupation; of enabling people to perform the occupations that foster health and well-being; and of enabling a just and inclusive society so that all people may participate to their potential in the daily occupations of life (Townsend&Polatajko, 2007).

The Declaration of Alma-Ata stated health, which is a state of complete physical, mental and social well-being, and not merely the absence of disease or infirmity, is a fundamental human right and that the attainment of the highest possible level of health is a most important worldwide social goal whose realization requires the action of many other social and economic sectors in addition to the health sector (WHO, 1978).

Question

Do you have any ideas to make your local community more inclusive?

Fundamental concepts

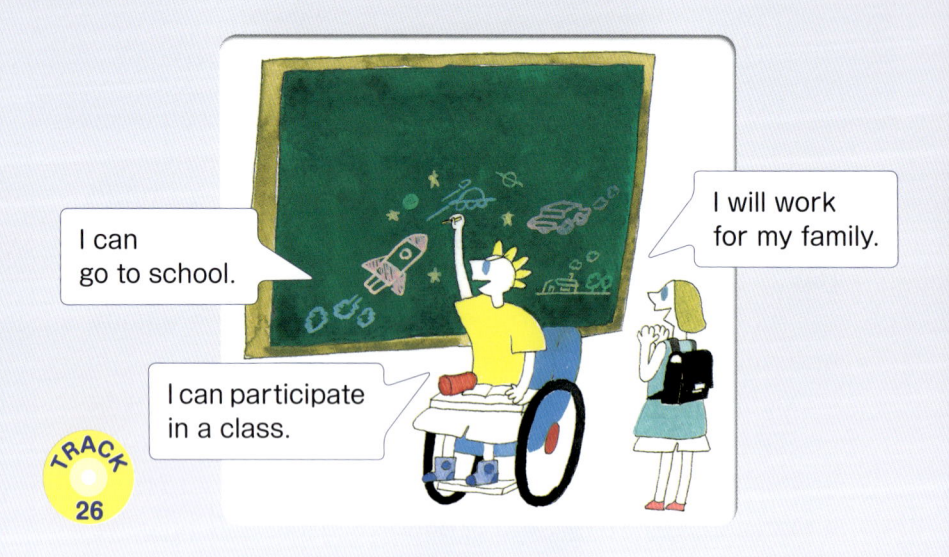

Section 5

Rehabilitation

Objective

To understand rehabilitation

Rehabilitation of people with impairments is a process aimed at enabling them to reach and maintain their optimal physical, sensory, intellectual, psychological and social functional levels. Rehabilitation provides disabled people with the tools they need to attain independence and self-determination.

§5 Rehabilitation

Taku: Ah...I got burnt last night while cooking.

Maki: Medically speaking, that's a thermal burn.

Taku: My right hand has lost function because of the pain and the bandage.

Maki: That is an impairment of body function.

Taku: I can't cook tonight.

Maki: That is activity limitation.

Taku: I'm sorry, but I can't be responsible at tonight's event as a team member.

Maki: That's participation restriction.

Taku: Can you help me?

Maki: Yes. You can use an environmental factor. I am a friend in the support and relationships category.

Taku: What are you talking about?

Maki: I am studying the ICF, International Classification of Functioning, Disability and Health, published by WHO in 2001.

Taku: Will you really help me at tonight's event?

Maki: Of course. No problem.

障害状態の表現

国際生活機能分類（ICF）は、多くの国や地域、異なる職種間における共通用語として開発された（WHO, 2001）。ICFは、生活機能の障害の種類や程度を表現する際にも便利である。タクが今夜のサークルの集まりで料理をする必要がなければ、タクの火傷は身体機能障害のみに留まるのだが、タクは料理をしなければならないので、活動制限を経験することになる。しかしマキという環境因子の助けにより、サークルという社会集団への参加制約を経験しなくてもよさそうだ。

Chapter 5: Fundamental concepts

Many people with disabilities who live in developing countries lack access to appropriate medical care and rehabilitation services. These people experience greater challenges in attaining and maintaining maximum independence and health than those living in developed countries.

Community-based rehabilitation (CBR) focuses on enhancing the quality of life for people with disabilities and their families, meeting their basic needs and ensuring inclusion and participation.

CBR guidelines were published by WHO in 2010. CBR has five key components: health, education, livelihood, social, and empowerment. All five components are incorporated during the implementation of CBR. The following CBR matrix is provided as an overview of CBR.

CBR:
リハビリテーションのための十分な設備も専門家もいない開発途上国では、地域に根差したリハビリテーション（CBR）が行われる。日本においても、山村など多くの地域で、CBRが有効となる。
1994年のCBRの定義では、障害者の能力の最大化が主な目的だったが、2004年に定義が改定され、リハビリテーションと機会の均等、ソーシャルインクルージョンを目標に、障害者、家族、団体、社会が合同で実行することになった（ILO, UNESCO, WHO）。
2010年に発表されたCBRガイドラインはWHOのウェブサイトから閲覧できる。

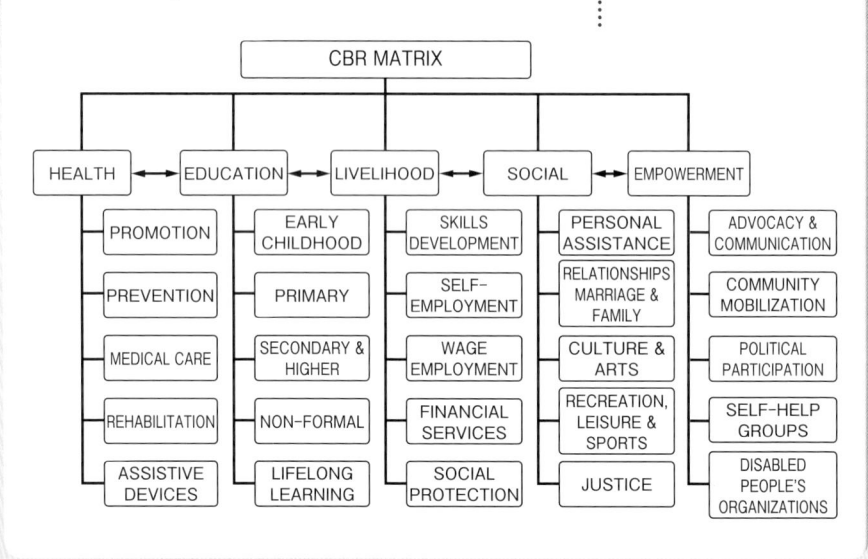

CBR MATRIX

HEALTH	EDUCATION	LIVELIHOOD	SOCIAL	EMPOWERMENT
PROMOTION	EARLY CHILDHOOD	SKILLS DEVELOPMENT	PERSONAL ASSISTANCE	ADVOCACY & COMMUNICATION
PREVENTION	PRIMARY	SELF-EMPLOYMENT	RELATIONSHIPS MARRIAGE & FAMILY	COMMUNITY MOBILIZATION
MEDICAL CARE	SECONDARY & HIGHER	WAGE EMPLOYMENT	CULTURE & ARTS	POLITICAL PARTICIPATION
REHABILITATION	NON-FORMAL	FINANCIAL SERVICES	RECREATION, LEISURE & SPORTS	SELF-HELP GROUPS
ASSISTIVE DEVICES	LIFELONG LEARNING	SOCIAL PROTECTION	JUSTICE	DISABLED PEOPLE'S ORGANIZATIONS

Rehabilitation

Occupational therapists are members of the rehabilitation team. The team works together to enable people with a disability to be as independent as possible. The Independent Living Movement and the idea of empowerment have motivated rehabilitation staff to rethink the goals in rehabilitation. The slogan, "nothing about us without us" is now used in events related to persons with disabilities.

There are differences in the medical and social view of disability. In the medical model, disability is seen as a deficiency or abnormality that should be normalized by professionals as much as possible. In the social model, disability is seen as arising from the interaction between the person and environment. Professionals who adopt a social view of disability believe that self-determination and empowerment are important goals in rehabilitation. Also, in the social model, persons with disabilities, their families, relevant organizations, professionals, and the society all work collaboratively to achieve these goals.

Question

Who needs rehabilitation? Where is the best place for rehabilitation?

Chapter 5

Fundamental concepts

TRACK 27

Exercise to lose weight!!

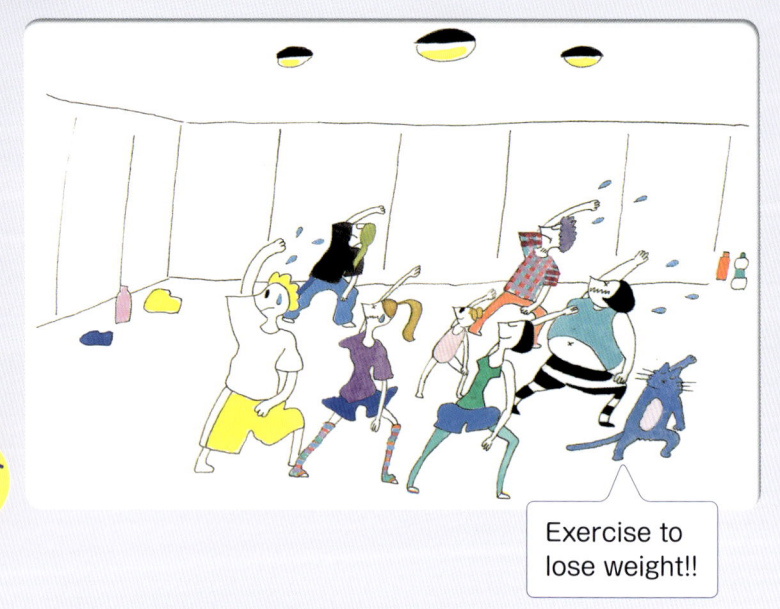

Section 6

Health promotion

Objective

To plan a project for your health promotion

In the medical model, health is considered as absence of symptoms or cure from disease. In health promotion, health is regarded as a resource for positive living, and it is maintained that all people can improve their own health by participating in health promoting occupations. Occupational therapists are experts in enabling people to participate in health promoting occupations.

§6 Health promotion

Maki : My mom is attending a health promotion program these days.

Taku : I've heard of those programs. People go walking, quit smoking, don't drink too much, and eat more vegetables.

Maki : She's learning how to organize her daily schedule. She's also making a post-retirement plan.

Taku : That sounds like occupational therapy.

Maki : Yes. An occupational therapist is one of the staff members in that program.

Taku : I thought occupational therapists work with people with disabilities.

Maki : Every human being is an occupational being. Occupational therapists are working for all people who need to promote health through occupation.

Taku : Do I need occupational therapy?

Maki : I'm not sure. But I recommend you check your occupational balance and to involve occupations linking to your future from an occupational perspective.

ヘルスプロモーション：1986年に世界保健機関（WHO）がオタワ憲章を発表してから、各国は住民の健康が維持されたり、より健康になるような保健政策を展開するようになった。日本が行っている健康日本21は、ヘルスプロモーションを目指したものである。栄養、運動、睡眠に気をつけ、健康的な生活習慣を送ることが疾病予防となる。また、安心できる安全な環境づくりも障害予防には欠かせない。
病気や障害を予防することだけがヘルスプロモーションではない。健康とは病気がないことだけを指すのではない。身体的、精神的、社会的により良い状態でいることができるように、住民と行政が協働して、より健康に暮らせる町づくりをしていく必要がある。

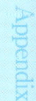

Chapter 5 Fundamental concepts

There are three strategies for health promotion in the Ottawa Charter (WHO, 1986)

Advocacy: Working with clients to raise critical perspectives, prompt new forms of power sharing, lobby or make new options known to key decision makers.

Enablement: Reducing differences in current health status and ensuring equal opportunities and resources to enable all people to achieve their fullest health potential. People cannot achieve their fullest health potential unless they are able to take control of those things which determine their health.

Mediation: Coordinated action by all concerned such as: governments, health, social and economic sectors, non-governmental and voluntary organizations, local authorities, industry and the media. Professional and social groups and health personnel have a major responsibility to mediate between differing interests in society for the pursuit of health.

アドボカシー（advocacy）は、唱道、代弁などと訳される。権利擁護という意味で使われることもある。当事者に力があれば、自ら主張していくことができるが、当事者が主張しにくい状況にある場合に、専門職などが当事者の立場から声を発し、行動していく。障害者の社会参加を促進するために、関連機関や関係者に対して働きかけるOTの役割は、アドボカシーである。

エネイブルメント（enablement）は、可能化、能力の賦与と訳される。当事者が能力を十分に発揮できるように機会や資源を確保することである。Enablementはdisablement（障害）の対語であり、できないところではなく、できるところに注目するときに使われる。なぜできないかではなく、どうしたらできるかを考えていくのである。

メディエーション（mediation）は、調停、仲介などと訳される。政府や関係団体など関連機関の連携がうまくいくように調整していくことである。地域でのネットワーク構築がこれにあたる。

§6 Health promotion

Health promotion

Health promotion in the Ottawa Charter is defined as the process of enabling people to increase control over, and to improve, their health. To reach a state of complete physical, mental and social well-being, an individual or group must be able to identify and to realize aspirations, to satisfy needs, and to change or cope with the environment. Health is, therefore, seen as a resource for everyday life, not the objective of living. Health is a positive concept emphasizing social and personal resources, as well as physical capacities. Therefore, health promotion is not just the responsibility of the health sector, but all organizations and groups responsible for promoting healthy life-styles and well-being (WHO, 1986).

Mary Reilly, a famous occupational therapist stated that "man, through the use of his hands as they are energized by mind and will, can influence the state of his own health (Reilly, 1962)". Reilly's idea is consistent with health promotion.

Question

How can you promote your health?

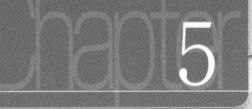

References

Canadian Association of Occupational Therapists. Enabling occupation: An occupational therapy perspective. Ottawa ON: CAOT Publications ACE, 1997.カナダ作業療法士協会著, 吉川ひろみ監訳, 作業療法の視点　作業ができるということ, 大学教育出版, 2000

Clark F, et al. Occupational science: Academic innovation in the service of occupational therapy's future. American Journal of Occupational Therapy, 45 (4), 300-310, 1991

Davis JA&Polatajko HJ. Occupational development. In Christiansen C&Townsend EA. Introduction to Occupation: The art and science of living, 2nd ed, pp. 135-174, Upper Saddle River, Pearson Education Inc, 2010

International Society for Occupational Science. The Way Forward Plan for ISOS, 2007. Retrieved from<http://shoalhaven.uow.edu.au/aosc/documents/isos_way_forward_july07.pdf> 1 March 2011.

Kielhofner G, Mallinson T, Forsyth K&Lai J. Psychometric properties of the second version of the occupational performance history interview (OPHI-II). American Journal of Occupational Therapy, 55 (3), 260-267, 2001

Kronenberg F, Algado SS, Pollard N. Occupational Therapy Without Borders: Learning From the Spirit of Survivors. Churchill Livingstone, 2005

Rawls J. A Theory of Justice, Cambridge, Mass, The Belknap Press of Harvard University Press, 1971.ジョン・ロールズ著, 矢島鈞次監訳, 正義論, 紀伊國屋書店, 1979

Reilly M. Occupational therapy can be one of the great ideas of 20th century medicine. American Journal of Occupational Therapy, 16 (1), 1-9, 1962

Stadnyk RL, Townsend EA, Wilcock AA. Occupational justice.

References

In Christiansen C&Townsend EA. Introduction to Occupation: The art and science of living, 2nd ed, pp. 329-358, Upper Saddle River, Pearson Education Inc, 2010

Townsend E. Occupational therapy's social vision. Canadian Journal of Occupational Therapy, 60 (4), 174-184, 1993

Townsend EA&Polatajko HJ ed. Enabling Occupation II. Ottawa ON: CAOT Publications ACE, 2007.エリザベス・タウンゼント, ヘレン・ポラタイコ編著, 吉川ひろみ, 吉野英子監訳, 続・作業療法の視点－作業を通しての健康と公正, 大学教育出版, 2011

Townsend EA&Wilcock AA. Occupational justice and client-centred practice: A dialogue in progress. Canadian Journal of Occupational Therapy, 71 (2), 75-87, 2004

United Nations (1948). Universal Declaration of Human Rights. 外務省, 世界人権宣言<http://www.mofa.go.jp/mofaj/gaiko/udhr/> アクセス日2011年3月1日

Wicks A. Understanding occupational potential. Journal of Occupational Science, 12 (3), 130-139, 2005

Wilcock AA. A theory of human need for occupation. Journal of Occupational Science, 18(1), 17-24, 1993

Wilcock AA. An occupational perspective of health, 2nd ed, Thorofare, SLACK Inc, 2006

Wilcock AA & Townsend EA. Occupational justice: Occupational terminology interactive dialogue. Journal of Occupational Science, 7 (2), 84-86, 2000

Whiteford G. Occupational deprivation: global challenge in the new millennium. British Journal of Occupational Therapy, 63 (5), 200-204, 2000

Whiteford G. Occupational deprivation. In Christiansen C&Townsend EA. Introduction to Occupation: The art and science of living, 2nd ed, pp. 303-328, Upper Saddle River, Pearson Education Inc, 2010

World Federation of Occupational Therapists (2009), Guiding Principles on Diversity and Culture.

World Federation of Occupational Therapists (2000), OTION.

<http://www.wfot.org/otion/> アクセス日 2011年3月1日
World Federation of Occupational Therapists (2010). Position paper: Occupational science. WFOT Bulletin, 61, 17.
World Health Organization (2001). International Classification of Functioning, Disability and Health (ICF).<http://www.who.int/classifications/icf/en/> アクセス日 2011年3月1日
World Health Organization (1978). Declaration of Alma Ata. Retrieved from<http://www.who.int/hpr/NPH/docs/declaration_almaata.pdf> アクセス日 2011年3月1日
World Health Organization (2010). Community-based rehabilitation guidlines<http://www.who.int/disabilities/cbr/guidelines/en/> アクセス日 2011年3月1日
World Health Organization (1986). Ottawa Charter for Health Promotion<http://www.who.int/healthpromotion/conferences/previous/ottawa/en/> アクセス日 2011年3月1日

Epilogue

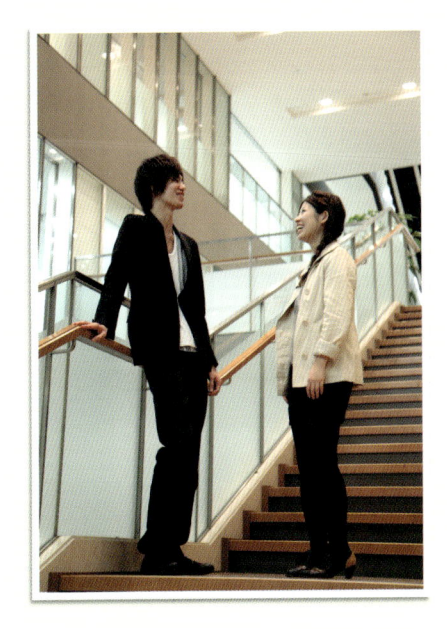

Finally, Maki and Taku have passed the national examination of occupational therapy in Japan.

Maki is working at a general hospital, and Taku is working with people with mental disorders.

Maki would like to be a candidate for the JICA program in the near future.

The Japanese welfare system

Services and Supports for Persons with Disabilities Act

In 2006, the Services and Supports for Persons with Disabilities Act was passed. The act introduced state measures that feature special change for PWDs(persons with disabilities), from protection to supports.

The main purposes of the act are

① To establish a universal platform of welfare services for all PWDs, mainly handled by local government
② To reform the welfare system in which PWDs can more easily use welfare services. And deregulation to maximize the utilization of limited social resources.
③ To foster and support the employment of PWDs with willingness to work and abilities.
④ To increase transparency and clarification concerning procedures and standards for fair services.
⑤ "Cost-sharing" in proportion to the quantity of services used. "Clarification" of the national government's fiscal responsibility.

The act was to be reviewed three years after passing. In 2009, a bill to revise the act was presented to the Diet.
For reference, see the Ministry of Health, Labor and Welfare.
<http://www.mhlw.go.jp/english/wp/policy/dl/02.pdf>

障害者自立支援法
平成17年法律123号　主な目的は障害者の自立に向けた支援である。主な関連法令は「身体障害者福祉法」「知的障害者福祉法」「精神保健福祉法」「児童福祉法」
改正障害者自立支援法が成立：平成22年12月3日

〈参考〉法務省　日本法令外国語訳データベースシステム
Japanese Law Translation 〈http://www.japaneselawtranslation.go.jp/〉
アクセス日　2011年3月1日

Long-term Care Insurance Law

In the 1960's, some policies of welfare for elderly people were initiated. In the 1970's, medical bills were free, but that led to increasing medical costs, so in 1982, elderly people began to bear part of their medical bills. In the 1980's, new issues emerged such as hospitalization of the bedridden and other patients with non-acute problems. In 1989, a 10-year plan for senior citizen health and welfare promotion was initiated, named the gold-plan. Then in 2000, Long-term Care Insurance was introduced.

Aims of Establishing Long-term Care Insurance

① To establish a system which responds to society's major concern about aging, the care problem, whereby citizens can be assured that they will receive care and be supported by society as a whole.
② Efficient delivery of a user-centered, quality long-term care service
③ Separate long-term care from medical care insurance, and establish a system as a first step towards revising the structure of social security

Ministry of Health, Labour and Welfare.2002
<http://www.mhlw.go.jp/english/topics/elderly/care/index.html>

介護保険法
平成9年法律123号　主な内容は介護保険とそのサービスについて。関連法令は「介護従事者等の人材確保のための介護従事者等の処遇改善に関する法律」「老人福祉法」「老人保健法」「医療法」「国民健康保険法」「国民年金法」

〈参考〉法務省　日本法令外国語訳データベースシステム
Japanese Law Translation 〈http://www.japaneselawtranslation.go.jp/〉
アクセス日　2011年3月1日

The Japanese welfare system

Act for the Mental Health and Welfare of Persons with Mental Disorders

In 1987, to improve treatment in mental hospitals, then the current Act on Mental Health was revised, and for the first time in Japan, rehabilitation into society was stated as the objective of the legislation. The name of the act was changed to Act for the Mental Health and Welfare of Persons with Mental Disorders in 1995. At the same time the purpose of "Promotion of independence and participation in socioeconomic activity" was added.

In relation to amendment of Services and Supports for Persons with Disabilities Act, some problems have been pointed out about the law.

Examples include the necessity for systematic review of existing laws that are related to mental health, lack of social resources, cost-sharing, and various problems concerning hospitalization service regulations for mental disease and guardians.

精神保健及び精神障害者福祉に関する法律
昭和25年5月1日法律第123号　目的は、精神障害者の医療・保護、その社会復帰の促進・自立と社会経済活動への参加の促進のための必要な援助、その発生の予防その他国民の精神的健康の保持及び増進により、精神障害者の福祉の増進・国民の精神保健の向上を図ることにある(1条より引用改変)。

名称の変更
「精神衛生法」1950年(上記参照)
　⇒「精神保健法」1987年7月施行
　⇒「精神保健及び精神障害者福祉に関する法律」1995年7月施行

〈参考〉法務省　日本法令外国語訳データベースシステム
Japanese Law Translation 〈http://www.japaneselawtranslation.go.jp/〉
アクセス日　2011年3月1日

Act on Employment Promotion etc. of Persons with Disabilities

In 1960, the Act on Employment Promotion etc. of Persons with Disabilities was passed and in 2005 and 2010 was amended. The purposes of the act are the stabilization and securing of employment for PWDs. There are three main measures. They are the obligation to employ a ratio of PWDs, payment at legal rates, and implementation of vocational rehabilitation.

Business owners must employ a certain number of PWDs as a proportion of all employees. For example, the ratio for private companies is 1.8 %. However, special subsidiary companies can be established and that can be counted in the employment of the entire corporate group. If a company can achieve the set employment ratio, the company gets 27000yen per person per month as employment adjustment subsides. But if it cannot, the company must pay 50000yen a month for the shortage of each person per month(Levy and Grant System). PDWs can receive occupational rehabilitation in some special facilities, for example, Hello Work, and so on.

Recently the government of Japan has been pursuing a strategy of "from welfare to employment". So PWDs are asked to go to work.

<http://www.mhlw.go.jp/bunya/shougaihoken/service/shurou.html>

障害者の雇用の促進等に関する法律　1960年7月25日 法律第123号
身体障害者雇用促進法　1960年
　1976 年改正　身体障害者雇用の義務化
　1987 年改正　「障害者の雇用の促進等に関する法律」
　1997 年改正　知的障害者の雇用も義務化
　2006 年改正　精神障害者(精神障害者保健福祉手帳所持者)及び短時間労働者も含まれる

〈参考〉法務省　日本法令外国語訳データベースシステム
Japanese Law Translation 〈http://www.japaneselawtranslation.go.jp/〉
アクセス日　2011年3月1日

Globalization

Study and work abroad

What is the biggest advantage of going abroad to study occupational therapy?

First is acquisition of language. Moreover, it is language ability at a level that can be used when working in the specialty.

Second is the possibility of obtaining the chance to work as an occupational therapist in other countries .

Third is the possibility to be able to work in fields different from Japan. For example, depending on the situation of each country, independent opening of clinics and consultations may be possible although, in general, they are not recognized as business forms of occupational therapy in Japan.

By the way, there is an advantage of studying abroad after receiving your occupational therapist's qualification in Japan. You can understand the content you have learnt more deeply and may go to graduate school. Above all, returning to Japan, it is possible to work at once as an occupational therapist.

WFOT (World Federation of Occupational Therapists)

The mission of the World Federation of Occupational Therapists (WFOT) is to promote occupational therapy as an art and science internationally.

WFOT began with formal discussions at a meeting of occupational therapists held in England in June 1951, at which there were 28 representatives from various countries. A Preparatory Commission was held in Liverpool, England in 1952, attended by representatives from seven countries with occupational therapy associations or organizations and written approval for the organization of such an association from three other countries. These ten associations from the USA, United Kingdom (England and Scotland), South Africa, Sweden, New Zealand, Australia, Israel, India and Denmark, inaugurated the WFOT.

In 1959 WFOT was admitted into official relations with the World Health Organization (WHO) and in 1963 it was recognized as a Non-Governmental Organization (NGO) by the United Nations (UN).

Quoted from <http://www.wfot.org/inside.asp>

WFOT Secretariat
PO Box 30 Forrestfield Western Australia Australia 6058

Globalization

JOCV (Japan Overseas Cooperation Volunteers)

Japan Overseas Cooperation Volunteers(JOCV) is an overseas volunteer dispatch program operated by an independent administrative agency, Japan International Cooperation Agency (JICA) under the jurisdiction of the Ministry of Foreign Affairs, as part of Official Development Assistance(ODA).

The recruitment age is from 20 to 39. Recruitment ranges over more than 100 professional categories. Of course, occupational therapy is one of them and contributes to, various practices for habilitation and rehabilitation of children and persons with disability, and various projects such as the development and establishment of social resources and systems in many countries.

See JICA <http://www.jica.go.jp/volunteer/>

JICA　独立行政法人国際協力機構
Japan International Cooperation Agency
〈http://www.jica.go.jp/volunteer/〉

Glossary

Activity of Daily Living (ADL) Activities for daily life involving taking care of oneself.

IADL Activities requiring interaction in the home and in the community.

Activity Choices The choice to engage during play and leisure.

Acute Very severe state, as in pain, disease, or some symptoms.

Adaptation Changing in response to new expectation or roles; making tasks simpler or less demanding to promote greater success.

Adult Day Care Programs that provide meaningful, structured activities for people with disabilities, and provide respite for primary care givers.

Agnosia Loss of ability to recognize familiar objects, for example, persons, sounds, shapes, or smells while the specific sense is not defective.

Americans with Disabilities Act (ADA) Legislation that provides civil rights to all individuals with disabilities; guarantees equal access and opportunity.

Arts and Crafts Movement An international design movement that originated in England and flourished between 1880 and 1910. It promoted use of fine arts and crafts to counter the alienation of industrialism.

Assessment Standardized processes, tools and instruments used for evaluation.

Assistive Technology Device(ATD) Tools, equipment and systems used to maintain or improve functional capacities of PWD.

Blood Pressure(BP) Circulating blood force against the walls of the arteries, veins and chamber of the heart.

Cerebral Palsy(CP) A motor function disorder caused by a permanent, nonprogressive brain lesion or d e f e c t from fertilization to 4 weeks after one's birth.

Cerebrovascular Accident(CVA) Injury to the brain caused by an interruption of the blood supply, also called stroke.

Clinical Reasoning Complex multifaceted cognitive process system that is necessary when practitioners plan intervention.

Clubhouse Model A rehabilitation program for PWD. Originating in the 1940's in New York, it developed from a mutual self-help group started by patients who had left mental hospital. The participants work in the business of the clubhouse while living in the locality and supporting each other.

Cognitive Disability Loss of mental ability across diagnostic categories; interferes with task behavior.

Collaboration To work together in a joint effort.

Community-Based Practice Intervention strategies that are focused on community in local life, and involve practices in local society.

Consultation To assist the consultee in reaching programmatic goals.

Coordination Combined activity of many muscles into smooth patterns and sequences of motion.

Create Interventions Approaches that focus on providing contextual and task experience.

Developmental Disability(DD) Atypical neurodevelopment loss or delay, with the onset occurring prenatally, perinatally,

or in early childhood.
Disability Limitation of activity as a result of impairment.
Disease Disorder indicating abnormality of mental or physical function.
Dynamic Splint Device composed of a molded splint base.
Empathy An attitude exemplified by an understanding of the feelings, and perspectives of another person.
Enabling Activities Therapeutic exercises that require involvement to clients but are not activities typically used in their culture.
Ergonomics Applied science of adapting the environment and other condition to the workers
Evaluation Measure and judge a specific function and the ability by using ongoing process and method.
Evidence-Based Practice A systematic process of using research to support clinical reasoning and practice dicisions.
Family-Centered Philosophy of service provision recognizing that families are the primary social context and receive care and intervention is based on the family's goals and values.
Feedback Information that learner receives about performance.
Frame of Reference Way to conceptualize and carrying out practice.
Function of Occupation Ways occupation influences function, development, adaptation, health, well-being, and quality of life.
Group Dynamics In occupational influence, relationships between individual, group and the environment.
Habits Automatic specific personal behavior on a day-to-day

basis.

Illness A state of poor health, which is sometimes considered as a synonym for disease or as the subjective perception by a patient.

Impairment Loss or abnormality of physiological, psychological, or anatomical structure or function and is a key factor for health professionals to determine appropriate treatment.

Independence Ability to know about oneself, to perform by oneself using self-responsibility and self-judgement.

Independent Living Movement It starts in the 1970's in the United States. The aim is for people, even with a high degree of disability to live in the community as they want.

Individualized Education Program(IEP) Education plan for children with disabilities focusing on individual function, and mandated by law in the United States.

Interviewing To share and understand experience and emotion by listening them carefully.

Job Site Analysis(JSA) Assessment used to define the essential demands of a job.

JOTA Japanese Association of Occupational Therapists.

Learning Disabilities(LD) Difficulty in learning. For example, reading or writing disorder, math disability etc, usually caused by brain-function or unknown factors.

Meaning of Occupation Significance of occupation in the individual context of real life, environment and culture.

Medical Model Approach based on medical method that focuses on the diagnosis and treatment of disease and injuries.

Moral Treatment In the 19th century, humanitarian approach to mental illness that centered around productive, creative and recreational occupations.

Narrative　Story that is created in a constructive format from a person's point of view, which describes a sequence of fictional or non-fictional events about an individual's life.

Occupation　All activity that humans need to live, for daily life, cultural values, self-care, work, enjoyment, and participation in the community.

Occupational Behavior　Characterization of development, habits, and roles relating to competence in occupational performance.

Occupational Choice　Process through which individuals commit and fulfil their occupational roles.

Occupational Competence　Ability to sustain occupational tasks.

Occupational Justice　From a social, political, economical view point, it is a state where individuals can meet their occupational needs and potential.

Occupational Role　Social expectation and behavioral enactment of activities and routines by individuals.

Occupational Science　Academic discipline studying occupation. (Chapter 5 参照)

Occupational Therapist　A graduate of an accredited occupational therapy program.

Performance Skills　Capacities and effectiveness related to observable elements of an action.

Physical Capacity Evaluation(PCE)　Assessment of physical and biomechanical aspects of the client's functional level. For example, active range of motion, muscle strength, posture, gait, sensation and cardiopulmonary status.

Play and Leisure Activities　Any activity providing pleasure, relaxation, and expression of creativity.

Profession A specialized knowledge-and skill-based specific education or training, which has been approved socially.

Public Health System of services for protection and improvement of community health by the organization of efforts combining preventive medicine, environmental approachs and social sciences.

Purposeful Activity Therapeutic activity that is selected to match the client's interests and which promotes specific outcomes.

Quality of Life State of well-being and functioning that includes level of comfort and enjoyment by participation in meaningful occupations.

Range of Motion(ROM) Arc of motion through which a joint passes.

Reasonable Accommodation Modification or adjustment that enables persons with disabilities to perform a task they are otherwise qualified to perform.

Risk Factors Factors interfering with growth, development or well-being including characteristics and behavioral tendencies of individuals, demographic variables, and environmental conditions.

Roles Behavioral expectations that accompany a person's occupied position or status in their society.

Socialization Acquisition of roles, attitudes, and behaviors consistent with the norms of the social group towards participation and adaptation.

Spirituality Fundamental and essential orientation of a person's life, that which inspires and motivates the individual.

Traumatic Brain Injury(TBI) Damage to the brain caused by an accident, fall, severe wound or other trauma.

Universal Design　Policy of designing environments and products so that they can be used by all people.

Wellness　A healthy lifestyle that includes nutrition, exercise, stress reduction, and other strategies.

『Willard & Spackman's Occupational Therapy Tenth Edition』を参考に作成

【監修者】
菊池恵美子（帝京平成大学　健康メディカル学部　作業療法学科長・教授／認定作業療法士，PhD）

【著　者】
山内ひさえ（作業療法士・保健科学博士）
吉川ひろみ（県立広島大学　保健福祉学部　作業療法学科長・教授／認定作業療法士，PhD）
Peter Kenneth Howell（県立広島大学　保健福祉学部　准教授／PhD）

【執筆協力者】
Alison Wicks（世界作業科学研究会会長／ウーロンゴン大学オーストラリアジアン作業科学センター所長）
姉崎祐治（英語会議通訳者）

【付属CD声の出演】
Kathleen Fukuhara／Laura Aoki／P. Sean Bramble／Paul Lishman／Peter Kenneth Howell

【CD収録】有限会社　写楽　　　　【イラスト】酒井はる

【デザイン】上村浩二　　　　　　【写真撮影】白石ちえこ

【写真撮影協力者】
池田浩二　菊池和美　下岡隆之　高橋瑞貴　露木雄太　根本悟子
久高優花　武藤真理　吉野望三

＊監修者・著者・執筆協力者の所属、職位は初版発行時のものです。

英語で学ぶ作業療法
Let's study OT in English

2011年3月25日	第1版第1刷
2015年3月30日	第1版第2刷
2016年5月20日	第1版第3刷
2023年2月10日	第1版第4刷Ⓒ

監　修　者　菊池恵美子
著　　　者　山内ひさえ
　　　　　　吉川ひろみ
　　　　　　Peter Kenneth Howell
発　行　人　小林俊二
発　行　所　株式会社シービーアール
　　　　　　東京都文京区本郷3-32-6　〒113-0033
　　　　　　☎(03)5840-7561　(代)　Fax(03)3816-5630
　　　　　　E-mail／sales-info@cbr-pub.com
　　　　　　ISBN 978-4-902470-70-3　C3047
　　　　　　定価は裏表紙に表示
装　　　幀　上村浩二
印刷製本　三報社印刷株式会社
　　　　　　Ⓒ Emiko Kikuchi 2011

本書の内容の無断複写・複製・転載は，著作権・出版権の侵害となることがありますのでご注意ください．

JCOPY ＜(一社)出版者著作権管理機構 委託出版物＞

本書の無断複製は著作権法上での例外を除き禁じられています．複製される場合は，そのつど事前に，(一社)出版者著作権管理機構(電話 03-5244-5088, FAX 03-5244-5089, e-mail: info@jcopy.or.jp)の許諾を得てください．